Blue Water, White Water

A True Story of Survival

D0873806

ROBERT C. SAMUELS

Blue Water, White Water

Robert C. Samuels

Published by Up The Creek Publishing
PO Box 335
Piermont, NY 10968

www.bluewaterwhitewater.com

Author Services by Pedernales Publishing, LLC.
www.pedernalespublishing.com

Author's note: I have tried to recreate events, locales and conversations from my memories of them. In order to maintain their anonymity in some instances I have changed the names of individuals and places, I may have changed some identifying characteristics and details such as physical properties, occupations and places of residence

Library of Congress Control Number: 2011939349

ISBN 978-0-9840194-1-0

Printed in the United States of America

For Karen Brown

Acknowledgements

The literary agent Flip Brophy was an early champion of this manuscript. I thank her for her efforts. I also thank Nancy Rosenfeld, another agent, for hers. Many writers encouraged me. Among those were, Joan Gussow and the late Joseph Heller. Tom Artin's proofreading help and editorial advice was invaluable.

Two others, Lucy Rosenfeld and John Dippel, were especially helpful, as was the editor and writer, Harvey Gardner. He was my late father's youngest pal and he is now my oldest. I treasure his wit, wisdom and advice.

December 2006

The evening is resplendent. It is a 70th birthday party for me and my friend, Charles Mouquin. We met when we were 12 years old, so this is not the first one we've celebrated together.

Some 20 people, mostly members of our families, are gathered in Charles's house, a Victorian mansion owned first by his grandparents. Charles and I are wearing tuxedos. I thought years from now my grandchildren might remember the evening as the night grandpa and his friend dressed up in those funny suits.

There are five grandchildren. Only Cassidy, the one and a half year-old daughter of my son Charlie and his wife Erin, is genetically connected to me. The other four are the grandchildren of my girlfriend Karen Brown. That doesn't matter. I've known and treasured them all since the day they were born.

I am a happy man. Karen is my love and we are devoted to each other. We share a beautiful house and we travel widely. Because I've had enough sense to follow Charles's advice (he's a semi-retired securities analyst), I am financially comfortable. We have many good friends. My health is fine. I stay busy with magazine assignments and local civic affairs.

A French restaurant is catering the meal. Waiters are serving champagne and hors d'oeuvres in the large living room with a tall Christmas tree in one corner. It is time for dinner. We enter a candlelit dining room aglitter with sparkling crystal and silver. I settle at my place at the table and switch off my power wheelchair.

December 1981

"When there's a bed open, we're going to move you down to the intensive care unit," the doctor says.

"When will that be?"

"It shouldn't be too long."

"Why do you want me there?"

"We want to watch you closely. We can do that better in the ICU."

"Oh."

He is matter-of-fact, calm, but so am I. I am stepping back and looking at this as I would an assignment. I am detached. I am covering my own story and I want to get it right. If it doesn't turn out to be something to write about, it certainly is something I'm going to talk about, maybe for years to come.

Being admitted to a hospital is a significant event in most lives. It certainly is in mine. It had happened to me only twice in my 44 years—once to have my tonsils out, and once for a broken wrist.

When I got up to use the bathroom early this morning I noticed a slight weakness in my left leg. I started to worry, but then I remembered all the yard work I'd been doing. "That's why the leg feels strange." I went back to bed and quickly fell asleep.

Six a.m. and the clock radio snaps on. The usual routine—my wife, Rikki, heads for one bathroom and I go to the other. The odd feeling in my leg surprises me until I recall the earlier trip to the bathroom. The leg is worse. I shower, shave and pause to tell Rikki about it. We agree that I probably pulled a muscle climbing the ladder to clean our roof gutters.

It's a little difficult going upstairs. I tell myself that if I ignore the weakness it will go away. Dressing is no problem, but going back downstairs is tricky. Fortunately, the house is very old and the stairs are narrow. I use the walls for support.

Rikki and I have our coffee and talk about other things. "Let me try the leg again," I suddenly say, walking to the sofa at the far end of the room. Something is definitely wrong— something serious. This isn't a pulled muscle. I've had those. This feels different from anything that's ever happened to me. Maybe I'm having a stroke.

"I'm calling Wanda. She'll know what to do," I say, sitting on the sofa. Wanda Heistand teaches nursing. Her husband, Dale, a good friend, is a Columbia University professor who had a very mild stroke not long ago. That's probably why I'm thinking about it.

I calmly tell Wanda my symptoms. As I talk, I look outside. It's a mild, overcast December morning. It is not a good day to die or to do anything else in particular. It's a real nothing day. Wanda is sympathetic and concerned. She doesn't mention the possibility of a stroke or try to guess what's wrong. She suggests I call a doctor. It's not yet seven am.

The problem is we don't have a family doctor since we're almost never sick. Then I remember that several months ago Rikki had strep throat and went to a young woman doctor who had recently opened a practice. In general, my wife is not crazy about doctors, but she liked this one, Dr. Julia Palmer. I'd said then that if I got sick I would also use Dr. Palmer.

I reach her answering service. I have a weakness in my left leg and it could be an emergency, I calmly report. No, I am not a patient but my wife is. The operator seems unimpressed. As I'm telling Rikki that I don't think we'll hear from Dr. Palmer, the phone rings. It's Dr. Palmer. She's very concerned. Go directly to the Nyack Hospital emergency room, she advises. No, she can't meet me because they haven't yet admitted her there to practice, but she'll call a colleague and he'll meet me. Good, I say, I don't have all day to spend on this; I have to get to work.

"You sure you want to drive?" asks Rikki. Yes, I want to drive. I always want to drive. We have two cars and I take the one with automatic transmission. I tell Rikki I don't believe my leg is strong enough now to push the clutch pedal on the other one.

During the first part of the short trip to the hospital I think about death, but I'm not frightened. The road is so familiar. I drive this way every morning on my way to work. The day again turns strange when I reach my usual entrance to the New York State Thruway and don't take it.

For the first time I tell Rikki that I think I may be having a stroke. As I say it, I wonder if I believe it. If I believe it, why am I driving on Route 9W, a dangerous highway? Am I play-acting? I honestly don't know. "You've given me a wonderful life," I say, as if it's over. Violins please, Mr. Previn.

Our mood is appropriately solemn as we reach the hospital parking lot. "Parking for Emergency Room Only," says the sign. Jesus, I suddenly think there is nothing wrong with my leg. I am a total asshole! When I get out of the car, though, I'm actually delighted to find the leg is weaker than before. For once, the car didn't fix itself on the way to the mechanic. I find I can't walk without a limp. I'm not making this up.

Dr. Palmer's colleague hasn't yet arrived. Instead, an emergency room doctor, ending his shift, examines me. He's an American in his late fifties and he looks exhausted. It's more than the long night that tires him, its life itself. He's a defeated man. Booze? Drugs? Bad marriage? Malpractice? Something got him. He takes a brief history. I tell him that I recently returned from a business trip around the world. I was in Sumatra. I was in New Delhi. Do I have a tropical disease? He's doubtful.

I remember a sophomoric joke from high school: "Doctor, Doctor, I'm suffering from a strange tropical disease."

"What's the disease?" asks the doctor.

"Lack o' nookie," replies the patient. I refrain from telling the joke. My temperature, heart rate and blood pressure are normal.

He tells me to lie on my back on an examining table with my knees bent. "Push your left foot into my hand. Now your right foot. Now again. I don't think your left leg is weak," he says, finally. "I can't find anything wrong. Why don't you go home."

"No," I tell him, "I'll wait for the other doctor." Rikki joins me in the curtained-off cubicle. We whisper.

"What if this new doctor also tells you there's nothing wrong?"

"Then we'll try another hospital. I know there's something wrong." Rikki has bought *The New York Times*. We split it and start to read; I can't concentrate. There's a sobbing child in the next cubicle who needs stitches; a victim of an auto accident in another.

I call work to let them know what has happened. "So

I'm going to be a little late," I tell Warren Jones, my boss and one of my best friends, as I hang up.

At last, Howard Long, the doctor Dr. Palmer has sent arrives. He's in his thirties—youthful, bearded, and self-assured. He listens carefully to my story and tests my legs. "Your blood pressure is normal. I don't think you're having a stroke but there is some weakness in your left leg. I'd like a neurologist to examine you."

Dr. Leon Schwartz, the neurologist, is an elegant dresser. I suspect the cuffs on his suit jackets actually button. His examination is quick. I lie on my back and push my feet into his hands. He tests my reflexes. They're normal. Doesn't everyone's leg jump when you hit it with a hammer?

I tell them about the trip. I've been back about a month. "Did you have shots before you left?" asks Dr. Schwartz.

"Yes. Typhoid, small pox and cholera, I think."

"Any upset stomachs, colds anything like that?"

"Yes, as a matter of fact I had stomach cramps and diarrhea over the Thanksgiving weekend." That was the weekend before last. "What do you think is wrong?"

"I'm not sure what you have, but I suspect it's Guillain-Barré syndrome. It's a neurological disorder that makes you very weak. We'd like to admit you and do some more tests." Dr. Schwartz seems like a man at the top of his game. He's in his forties, old enough to have all the necessary experience, but not yet tired of the job. I trust him.

They have me undress and don a hospital gown. A nurse folds everything neatly and slips it into a clear plastic bag. She gives it to Rikki to bring home. "That doesn't make any sense," I protest. "I won't be here all that long. Why don't I keep my clothes?"

"You don't know how long you'll be here," the nurse says. "Your wife can bring clothes in when you're discharged."

For the first time it occurs to me that I might not be home in a few hours.

It's already afternoon. Rikki needs to phone some of her skating students and do some household chores. I'm to call when I know my room number. She'll be back in a couple of hours.

An elderly hospital volunteer is pushing me on a stretcher. It makes me feel silly "You're heavier than you look," he says.

"Yeah, I know," I say sharply. I hate nothing more than discussing my weight. I weigh about 190, up from the 178 I'd reached several months ago after strenuous dieting. Before that, I'd been around 230 and that wasn't my all-time high. I am exactly six feet tall and always look as though I weigh less than I do. At 190, I feel I don't look bad.

My bed is by the window on the backside of an upper floor of the hospital's new wing. It looks across the highway at a cemetery that rises steeply up a hill. Tombstones and monuments bearing the family names of people I've lived with much of my life fill the place. The hospital faces Nyack High School. I graduated from there in 1955. I have lived in and near Nyack since 1949. My roots are here.

My roommate is an Italian-American in his seventies who nods hello when I arrive then quickly dozes off. I gaze out the window. I'm tired of this whole business. I want to go home.

When my roommate's wife and son visit, I try the paper again, but I can't avoid their conversation. "You should be happy,' Pop," the son tells him, "The doctor said you're going to be all right." Pop looks anything but happy.

"Everyone is asking about you," his wife adds. "They're glad you're coming home." She's at least ten years younger than he is. The son is about my age and sloppy fat.

The son starts a conversation with me. He lives in Connecticut where he's a manager in a Sears, but he grew up in Haverstraw. His parents still live there. Nyack and Haverstraw were bitter sports rivals when we were in high school. He was on the Haverstraw football team. Do I remember the Nyack teams? Sure I do. Do I remember two Nyack players from that era who went on to play in the National Football League? Is the Pope Catholic? "What are you in for?" he asks.

"The doctors want to do some tests. They think I may have Guillain-Barré syndrome. Ever hear of that?" His pleasant face is suddenly troubled. "What's wrong?" I ask, frightened.

"A buddy of mine was laid up in the hospital three months with that, but he's better now." That can't be, I think. I don't have three months to spend in a hospital.

"But three months," I say.

"Yeah, I know. Maybe you don't have it so bad," he says. Maybe I don't have it at all, I think.

"Tell me all about your friend."

"A whole bunch of us were down in Acapulco on vacation. The day before we were to come back, he felt very weak. We practically had to carry him on the plane. As soon as we landed, we took him right to a hospital. He had a rough time, but he's better now." He looks at his watch. It's time for him to leave.

"Pop, I have to go. After I drop Mama home, I have that long drive home but just think, next time I'll see you, you'll be home," he says, bending awkwardly to kiss his father.

"Ralph, Ralph," the old man says.

"Yes, Papa."

"Lose some weight, Ralph."

"I plan to Pop, just as soon as the holidays are over.

There are so many parties and such good food. I'll start right after." I feel Ralph's pain and humiliation but I think Ralph could start before the holidays. After all, it's only December second.

I'm supposed to call Rikki. I reach for the bedside phone and find that my hand is too weak to pick it up. I can't believe how feeble I've become. I'm not frightened. I think it's funny.

I want the back of the bed up so I can read the paper but the control has slid down the railing, out of my reach. I call a nurse to help me. "Why would anyone put the control down there?" I ask.

"To torture patients," she says with a wink. Only a short while ago I could have reached it easily. I find I only can read the stories at the bottom of the front page because the paper is too heavy to move. Again, I think it's funny.

When Rikki arrives she's annoyed with me for not calling her. She is one of world's most reliable people and doesn't easily tolerate missed calls and appointments. If you asked her to meet you on the south walkway of the Golden Gate Bridge at noon on July 4 ten years from now and she wasn't there, you'd assume she was dead. As a competitive figure skater, she'd had to show up on time for lessons or catch absolute hell from her coach.

I explain that I'm too weak to pick up the phone. I try it again, so she can see. I still can't. I also repeat Ralph's story about his friend. Then I show her how heavy the newspaper has become. "I'm turning into the world's weakest man."

"You better watch it or I'll knock you into next week," Rikki threatens. We laugh like fools.

Now Dr. Schwartz and Dr. Long arrive with Dr. Peter Fields, an internist. They don't seem surprised when I tell them how much weaker I've become. They ask Rikki to wait outside. Dr. Schwartz wants to inject my leg with something.

"If it is another disease with the same symptoms," he explains, "you'll immediately start to regain your strength."

"That sounds like the princess kissing the frog. You know, like something in a fairy tale. That sort of thing," I say. They smile tensely and Dr. Schwartz gives me the shot in the left thigh. Nothing happens. Now Dr. Fields, who is a respiratory specialist, has me blow as hard as I can into a metal device.

"We'd like to do a lumbar puncture," says Dr. Schwartz.

"What's that?"

"It's also called a spinal tap."

"I don't want it."

"We really need this test."

"Is it so important?" I ask.

"It's vital. It'll measure the protein level of the fluid in your spinal cord. It's the one way we have of determining for sure if you have Guillain-Barré," Dr. Schwartz explains.

"Why don't you want it, Bob?" asks Dr. Fields, his balding forehead wrinkled with concern.

"I'm afraid of it. I've read it's dangerous and painful."

"It is really a routine procedure," Dr. Fields says, reassuringly. "As for the pain, you'll use extra Novocain, won't you, Leon?"

"Sure," says Dr. Schwartz.

They are the doctors. There is no way for me to argue with them unless I'm willing to be totally unreasonable and unscientific. I agree to the spinal tap.

"I don't think I ever heard of Guillain-Barré," I tell Dr. Schwartz when we're alone.

"I bet you have," he says. "Remember in 1976 people got sick from swine flu inoculations. What they had was Guillain-Barré. There was a great deal of publicity about it then." Now I remember. It paralyzed some people.

"Dr. Schwartz, if you were me," I ask, "would you rather have a stroke or Guillain-Barré?" I am thinking about my friend Dale, the Columbia professor. He was in the hospital for less than a week when he had his stroke, not three months.

"Guillain-Barré, no doubt about it."

"Why?"

"Because you recover completely from Guillain-Barré. Strokes usually leave some terrible aftereffects."

I'm confused. The only aftereffect Dale suffered was some slight restriction in the movement of one thumb. I have read a great many popular books and articles about medicine and the life of doctors, and now, when it counts, I can't remember one helpful fact.

Before I have a chance to ask another question, Dr. Schwartz has me turn on my side and he injects the Novocain somewhere above the small of my back. After a short while, the area goes numb. Now he's ready for the spinal tap itself. He's got me bent as much as possible on my side. There's terrific pressure against my back as he forces the needle between my vertebrae and into my spinal column. I feel no pain but I'm ill, nauseated. I'm glad it's over. I hope I never have another. That's when he tells me that they want to move me to intensive care.

Rikki and I are holding hands as I give her a report on everything that's happened. She knows even less than I do about spinal taps and strokes. We share a sense of entering an alien world.

"Some real friends ordered this for you," jokes the nurse as she delivers my dinner tray. It has only ice cream, milk, and coffee on it. I haven't eaten all day, but I don't care what they serve me. I'm still queasy from the spinal tap. My hand can barely hold the spoon. The ice cream is half melted and tastes grainy. I sip some of the milk through a straw. It's been years since I had milk this way.

I ask Rikki to find a nurse. I need to pee but I know I'm too weak to walk to the bathroom without help. The nurse tells me to use a urinal. She draws the curtain between the beds and she and Rikki step out. I'm inhibited. If I could hear some water running it might help. She can't do that. "Could you bring me a basin of warm water for me to put my hand in?"

"What good will that do?"

"In the Air Force, sometimes when someone was sleeping we put their hand in warm water. It made them wet their beds."

"Why don't you try the urinal again?"

When she draws the curtain again, I think of a Colorado mountaintop I visited this spring while getting material for some stories. Water from melting snows gushed down the mountain with a tremendous roar. Someone told me that they film beer commercials there. These watery thoughts don't help.

"I guess I didn't have to go so bad," I say when Rikki returns. I'm lying.

"Have you gone since you've been here?" she asks.

"Well, no."

"Darling, that's been all day."

"You know how I am. I don't go often. I'll go later."

"Mr. Samuels?"

"Yes." It's a very young, attractive nurse with a clipboard.

"I have to ask you some questions."

"Sure, but tell me what's happened to my bed in intensive care?" Am I the first patient ever to be in a hurry to get to the ICU?

"I guess it's not yet ready."

"Are we waiting for someone to die to free it?"

"You're terrible," she says, but her tone suggests I may be right.

I've already answered most of the questions on her form. Again I tell about childhood diseases and family mortality. My mother died of stomach cancer when I was a small child, and my older sister died of a brain tumor in 1975. My father is alive and well and, at 79, living in Mexico, I say with relief.

Finally, they've come to get me. Several months ago I had visited my mother-in-law in the intensive care unit of a hospital in Port Chester, New York. She had suffered a mild heart attack. The ward was a large, cheerful room with a distant view of Long Island Sound.

The elevator descends and they roll me into Nyack's ICU. It's a tomb, a bunker. If it's not in the basement or sub-basement, it might as well be. This grim place has no windows. The center of the ward has a nursing station with desks and equipment. Around the perimeter are a dozen beds with patients, all seemingly hooked to machines. Thank God, I need no machines.

My doctors are standing by the one empty bed. They look like hosts waiting for the overdue guest of honor. "Sorry I'm late fellas," I say cheerily as two nurses slide me from the stretcher to the bed. Dr. Long laughs politely and the others smile.

"How are you feeling now?" Dr. Long asks.

"Fine."

"Any problems?"

"No, none at all."

"He hasn't been able to urinate," blurts Rikki. I'd almost forgotten that. Now, as she mentions it, I again have to go badly.

I think my problem is psychological, not physical, I say.

"When did you last go?" asks Dr. Long.

"When I got up this morning." The doctors exchange glances.

"The reason you haven't been able to urinate is physical, not psychological," says Dr. Long. "I think he should have a catheter," he casually tells the others. They nod in agreement, and I nod too, as if I also think it a splendid idea. Actually, I'm nodding in terror.

I remember visiting my father in a Manhattan hospital some 10 years ago, just after his prostate operation. It was early evening on a steamy August day, and I was on my way home from work as a reporter at the *World-Telegram and Sun*.

In the dim room light, I thought my father was dead. Then I saw he was breathing but asleep. Through the open fly of his pajamas I could see his penis, a stainless steel catheter stuck in its end. The shock of seeing that catheter in my father is still with me. For a long while the memory gave me nightmares. Every time I hear the word prostate I think of that catheter. Now, they want to give me one.

I am speechless with fright. They draw the curtain around my bed and ask Rikki to leave for a few minutes. She has no idea of my terror. I had never told her about the catheter in my father. I'd never told anyone.

It turns out that something I had secretly feared for 10 years is nothing to fear at all. The procedure is quick and painless. It is a great relief to have it over, but mostly it's a relief to urinate. It's the true pause that refreshes.

They're going to leave the catheter in, they explain, because it will be impossible for me to urinate for a while. The nerves to the muscles that control the bladder have stopped working. I don't care, as long as no one sees the catheter. No one else should have my nightmares.

"Are you sure I have Guillain-Barré?" I ask Dr. Schwartz.

"Almost certain. The protein level of your spinal fluid is very high."

"Do you know how I got this disease?"

"No, not positively. It may have been an allergic reaction to the inoculations you had before your trip. Then again, many cases report upper respiratory infections or stomach flu before coming down with it. You said you had stomach problems over Thanksgiving," he points out.

For the first time he explains what's going on inside my body: "Your nerves have a fatty covering called myelin. It acts as an insulator. With Guillain-Barré, this insulation is burned away and messages sent from your brain to your muscles are short-circuited. As a result, your brain isn't able to tell your muscles what it wants."

"When will it stop? How far will it go?"

"We can't tell," he says, "but one thing for you to remember is that eventually the myelin grows back and you do recover."

They've hooked electrodes to my chest. My heart rate and other information are displayed on a digital readout. There are tubes and wires all over me. Every time the slightest thing goes wrong with one of these devices, an alarm rings. They go off so often that no one seems upset when they hear one. I wonder what happens when there's a genuine emergency.

Dr. Fields again has me blow hard into an instrument. You're having trouble breathing," he declares. I don't feel I am at all, but what do I know? He wants me to use a respirator. Although I can breathe on my own now, I may have real problems later on, he says.

Rikki and I know almost nothing about respirators. All I can remember is that my friend, Stanley Spiegel, was on one for some hours following open-heart surgery. They'd shoved something down his throat and when they removed it he was left with a terrible sore throat.

Why don't you go get some dinner now, the doctors tell Rikki. They'll put me on the respirator while she's gone. Somehow they neglect to mention that I won't be able to talk when she returns. We have no last words.

"Why not use an iron lung?" I ask after she's gone. I remember all the dramatic newsreels I'd seen as a kid of polio victims in iron lungs. It would be a way to avoid that sore throat. It had sounded terrible.

Iron lungs are old fashioned, Dr. Fields explains. They're seldom used today. Respirators are better. What do I know? My ignorance is vast.

The procedure is quite simple. They are going to spray my throat with some fluid from an aerosol can. That'll keep me from gagging. Then they'll shove this thick tube down that will be hooked with a hose to the respirator. It doesn't occur to me to ask how, with the tube in my throat, I'll eat, drink, talk, or even spit.

Now it's happening. They've sprayed my throat. Dr. Fields is pushing the thing in. Christ, no wonder Stanley had a sore throat. This hurts like hell but the spray works—I'm not gagging. Did Linda Lovelace use it in the movie "Deep Throat?" The tube is surely larger than anything Linda had to swallow. What kind of mind do I have?

I'm choking. Jesus! A nurse has a thin, clear, plastic tube and she's suctioning mucus from my mouth and my nose. The plastic tube steals my breath, making my extremities tingle from lack of oxygen. When she jams the catheter down my throat, I feel as if I'm gagging, except I cannot gag. When she pushes it up my nose, my eyes tear and the irritation makes my nose run even more. I'm a damn fountain of mucus!

"Relax, let the machine breathe for you," says Dr. Fields. That's easy for you to say, but it's not so easy to do. I'll try. One breath, two breaths. I can't do this—it's impossible. The machine has a rhythm that is its rhythm not my rhythm. It has a sound that's all its own too. It's the noise of a bellows driven by a powerful electric motor.

Again, I'm choking. More suctioning. I'm drowning. How long are they going to keep this tube in? I haven't asked. Can't ask now. Don't think about that.

"Relax, Bob, relax," Dr. Fields is saying. "The machine will breathe for you." I'm drowning again. More suctioning. My nose is a river.

I'm so uncomfortable. All I can move are my arms, one leg and my head—that's all. The rest is too weak. I want to turn over but I can't. "I'm going to put you on your side," says the nurse who has been suctioning me. Sweet Angel, how did you know? She rolls me to my left, skillfully stuffing pillows behind me so I don't slide back. Comfort, relief, but now I'm drowning again. More suctioning—nose, mouth. I'm a fucking fountain of mucus!

I hear Rikki's voice over the sound of the respirator, but I can't see her yet. Now she's here and she looks stunned. She didn't know what it meant when they said they were putting me on a respirator. I can't tell her that I feel all right now, now that she's back. Because of the tube, I can't talk. Instead, I wink.

"Oh darling," she says, clutching my hand, her eyes brimming with tears.

~

My mouth fills with more mucus than I can swallow. My nose runs and the machine sounds a dreadful honk. Rikki is pushed aside by a nurse who quickly stops the awful noise and suctions me. More alarms go off—they're always going off. Are they mine? Does anyone know? Does anyone care?

The nurse, in her rush, neglects to close the curtain. So Rikki sees the suction tube jammed in my mouth, then in each nostril. Her face contorts with the effort to hide her anguish. I want to tell her that it's okay—that things are not as bad as they look. I want to hold her in my arms to comfort her. Instead, I wink again. I cannot speak. I am totally mute.

She holds my hand. "The doctors say you'll make a full recovery. You know you'll make a full recovery." It is more of a plea than a statement, but I nod my head in agreement. I need no reassurance. I know I will recover.

"Do you want me to stay all night?" I shake my head no. She looks exhausted. Her blue eyes seem dull with worry; her blonde hair looks lank. She's a trim, athletic woman, normally full of pep but this has been a long day. What would be the point of her staying?

"There are no visiting hours in this part of the hospital," she tells me. "You can come when you want and stay as long as you want. I can stay." I vigorously shake my head no! I want her to take care of herself. She is my love.

Again, the flood of mucus is overwhelming me. "Nurse! Nurse!" Rikki cries. An Indian nurse comes in and starts opening the clear plastic box, containing the suctioning material. Hurry, please, hurry. I'm drowning again. Look at her! She's taking her bloody, sweet time opening the fucking box. It's as though it holds something precious.

She asks Rikki to leave, then closes the curtain.

I can't stand this. Jesus! Finally, she's suctioning my mouth. Oh, thank God! Oh, the relief! Wait a minute you dumb bitch, what about my nose? Don't leave. You forgot to suction my nose. I try to lift an arm to point to my nose, but

I can't. I don't have the strength. I try to stop the respirator, to breathe against it, but it is too powerful for me.

Rikki is back. I want to show her something is wrong. I shake my head—I move my leg. Jesus, do something please. "Nurse, nurse!" she cries again. I'm swallowing gallons of mucus. The stuff covers my upper lip. Alarms are sounding somewhere.

The Indian nurse responds. "What's wrong, darling?" she asks. Her voice is so sweet, her touch so gentle. My nose you bitch! My fucking nose! "Do you know what's wrong?" she asks Rikki.

"His nose is running terribly."

"Oh, yes, I see," she says gently. "I suction." Again, Rikki must leave and the curtain is drawn. Everything this nurse does is slow fucking motion, slower than the beat of the respirator. She opens the box. She dons the gloves. She inserts the suction catheter into the vacuum tube. Now she's suctioning my nose. "There darling, isn't that better?" she asks me, throwing away the catheter and her gloves. No bitch, my nose is fine but now my mouth needs suctioning.

"Your husband is okay now," she tells Rikki as she leaves. But I'm not okay. My mouth is full again. I can't swallow all this stuff. I can't. I shake my arms and my leg as much as I can to signal Rikki. Again Rikki calls for a nurse. This time we get a young girl. Quickly, she suctions both my mouth and nose. Some difference!

Rikki is reluctant to leave but Dr. Fields is telling her that she should go and I nod in agreement. Now the Indian nurse is stroking my head and talking to Rikki. She says her name is Doria. "I take good care of your husband tonight. Don't worry. I take good care. Go home and rest."

Rikki wants more. She wants to establish some human contact with this nurse. "Are you Indian?" she asks.

"Oh yes I am." Doria's voice is a singsong.

"My husband was in India recently and he loved it." I didn't love it but it fascinated me. I know Rikki is trying to give the nurse a reason to like me.

"Where was he?" They're talking about me as if I'm not here.

"Bombay." Oh, no, it wasn't Bombay. It was New Delhi. I'm shaking my head no as hard as I can but they don't notice.

"How long was he there?"

"Just one day but he visited the Taj Mahal. He loved that." Oh, Jesus, Rikki, you can't visit the Taj from Bombay in a day.

"Are you sure he was in Bombay?" asks Doria. She realizes there is a geographical error.

"It was Bombay, wasn't it darling?" I shake my head no so very weakly.

"New Delhi?" Doria questions. I shake my head yes and mucus spills from my mouth and nose. She asks Rikki to leave and again the curtain is closed. This time she suctions both my mouth and nose, but it's slow.

Now Rikki is back. "I fly to New Delhi tomorrow," Doria tells Rikki. "I go home for a holiday with my husband and baby." I'm overjoyed by the news.

"Oh, that's too bad," says Rikki. "After tonight you won't be able to take care of Bob." Has Rikki lost her mind?

"I come back in a month. I take care of him then. Don't worry." Doria says. I'm outraged. A month! I won't be here in a month. How can she think I'll be here in a month?

"Bob won't be here in a month," says Rikki in a shaky voice. "He'll be better." Of course I will.

"I hope so," says the nurse, "but if he's here, I take care of him."

I don't have enough strength now to push the call button.

They've rigged a string to it so I can pull it to call a nurse. The first time I try, I find I'm too weak to do even that.

Rikki realizes that isn't going to be a way for me to summon help during the night. Doria promises to check me frequently. Rikki says I should twist my left leg vigorously if I need help. It's the only part of me I can still move with any strength. "Don't worry," says Doria.

Will Rikki ever go? "You'll be all right. Doria will take good care of you." She is trying to reassure herself. "Are you sure you want me to go?" she asks again. I nod yes. "I could stay. I could spend the night," she pleads. I nod no.

It is pointless. She needs sleep. The dog has to be walked, usually my job, and fed, her job. There will be phone calls on the answering service about skating lessons—orders at the post office for our mail order business. To the rest of the world this has been an ordinary day.

"Good night darling," Rikki says, fighting away tears. "I love you." I cannot respond. "You love me, don't you?" she asks. I nod my head. God, do I ever! I watch her go.

I need suctioning. I twist my leg violently. Where the fuck is Doria? I hear the sound of my respirator. Alarms are beeping all over. The bells are ringing for me and my gal. There is mucus running from my nose and mouth. Why did I let Rikki go? How will I get help? I twist my leg as hard as I can. Maybe someone will come. I see nurses passing, but no one notices my turning leg. I swallow more mucus. Now there's a bell ringing near me. It's one of my alarms. A nurse comes to check, to turn it off and sees I need suctioning. Finally, relief!

There is a night in this tomb. As the hour grows late, they turn off some of the lights, but it is nowhere near dark. It grows quieter, but it is nowhere near silent. The public address system stops paging doctors. I hear my respirator if I listen for it, but already it has become part of my life. Its rhythm is now my rhythm. Could I breathe without it? I don't know. Alarms ring and nurses move about. The sound of something going kerplunk comes from the nurses' station. Because I am lying down and can't move my head, my visibility is very limited.

"Mr. Samuels?" asks a young, bearded doctor. I try to answer but of course, I can't make a sound. Doria materializes from somewhere and confirms that I am indeed Mr. Samuels.

"Mr. Samuels, my name is Davis. I'm a resident here. I'm supposed to give you a nose tube so you can be fed while on the respirator. Do you understand?" I try to nod but I discover I can no longer even do that. I can't respond. "Mr. Samuels, blink your eyes if you understand." I blink. "Mr. Samuels, I have to give you the tube because you can't eat normally while on the respirator." I blink again.

They put up the back of the bed, which pitches my head forward. Mucus pours from my mouth and nose. "Nurse, Mr. Samuels needs suctioning," says Dr. Davis.

For a change, Doria hustles. She's afraid of the doctor. She pushes my head back and it hits something with a conk. It is strange to hit your head and not be able to rub it. A sensor rips off my chest and an alarm sounds. She puts the sensor back. Now I feel a pull at my penis. Something has snagged the tube attached to the catheter and pulled it out. No alarm-sounds for this and there is no way for me to tell them. But all I really care about is lying down again. Sitting up is incredibly uncomfortable. Hurry, please hurry!

Under the glare of a strong light, Dr. Davis slips the plastic tube up my right nostril. He works smoothly and easily. "I have to be sure you have this thing in your stomach and not in one of your lungs. That could cause real problems," he says.

The nose tube is in place. He attaches a rubber bulb to its end and places his stethoscope against my stomach. Then he squeezes the bulb. I feel my stomach rumble. "It's in the right place all right," he says. "I can hear it. You're all set."

He senses my discomfort and quickly gets Doria to help him put me back on my side and get me settled. Oh Lord, sweet relief! He's gathering his stuff to leave. He doesn't know about the catheter! I'm blinking like crazy, trying to get his attention.

He notices. "What's wrong? Something's bothering you, isn't it?" I blink once. He looks around the bed and spots the problem. "Jesus," he swears softly, "one of us pulled out your catheter. "Thanks for letting me know." I blink again, trying to say you're welcome.

The catheter is back in place. Dr. Davis has gone. I miss him. He'd talk with me and I'm lonely. No one is around. Things are quiet—quiet as they ever get. I hear just an occasional kerplunk from the nurses' station. I know that noise. What the hell is it? There's some white stuff flowing through the nose tube into my stomach. I taste nothing. I'm not being fed, I'm being filled.

The nose tube has set off a fresh eruption of mucus. The alarm sounds. It's insistent. Doria responds, she suctions, the mucus flows, the alarm sounds, Doria comes, she suctions. On and on it goes. Just when it seems it will never stop, never even slow, it does slow.

Time passes. I think of my father and my stepmother in Cuernavaca, Mexico. They found the ideal place to retire. They have such a nice life there. Jesus, it would kill my father if he knew where I am.

Suctioning, I need suctioning. How the fuck does this happen so quickly? One minute I'm fine, the next I'm drowning. I twist my leg but it only moves a little. The myelin must be burning away there too. "The lights are going out all over Europe," said Winston Churchill at the beginning of World War II. Now, the lights are going out all over me.

Where the fuck is Doria? I'm going to die before she comes. Oh, Jesus! "Medic! Medic!" they yell in war novels. I can't call—I can't even whisper. That dumb goddamn fucking Indian cunt! Get your fucking ass over here! Jesus, this thing is making me a racist sexist, a delightful combination. It's so damn difficult to breathe. I say, Doria darling, while you're up, get me suction.

The loud respirator alarm is sounding. She can't ignore that goddamn thing. It'll wake the dead. Who knows, in this ward maybe there really are dead to wake. "Where is Doria?" asks a young nurse. "I wish I knew where Doria disappears to," she sighs after suctioning me. "Let me look at you." She peers down, brown eyes moist and sympathetic. "You're Mr. Samuels, I heard about you. You're sick now but you're going to make a complete recovery." You're fucking A right, baby, fucking A! You're my kind of nurse.

"You're a mess," she tells me sweetly. "You need a bath. Doria should do it but I don't know where she is but I'll clean you up. We can't leave you this way." She draws the curtains around my bed and brings a basin of warm water, washcloths and towels. Now she pulls back the bedclothes and, with gentleness, strips my hospital gown, all the while talking to me. Her name is Jenny, she tells me. She's been a nurse since June when she graduated from Rockland Community College. She is getting married in the spring.

Jenny loves working in the ICU, enjoys the twelve-hour shifts, and the time off. I adore her. All the while she's talking she's washing my body. She touches me gently where no one but lovers have touched me since I was a child. Although she is young and very attractive, there is nothing sexual in this.

Even so, her touch is personal. She's not washing a car and she knows it.

I smell the Ivory soap and, as always, the odor brings back memories of my mother. She had bathed with Ivory too. I remember that although I was just in kindergarten when she died during an operation for stomach cancer.

Many primitive peoples believe that as long as someone remembers you, you are still alive. Although I reject the mystical and have no belief in a hereafter, I think there is an undeniable truth to this.

So, because of my hazy memories, my mother lives again and again. Some of the things that evoke her for me—her monuments—are Ivory soap and her favorite foods, corn on the cob, coffee ice cream and lamb chops. They say she had a marvelous sense of humor. I think those things would have made her laugh.

Before Jenny can get a fresh gown on me, I need suctioning. As she starts to do my mouth, Doria pushes through the curtains. "What are you doing with my patient?" she demands in a voice that whines into an indignant squeal.

"You weren't around and he needed suctioning," says Jenny, a little defensively.

"What happened to his gown?"

"He also needed to be washed. He was a mess."

"I'll take care of my patients. You take care of yours!"

"Fine with me," says Jenny, whirling on her heel, and pushing out of the cubicle.

Doria stuffs my arm through the sleeve of the gown. She's angry and rough. Electrodes pop off my body, an alarm sounds. "You are my patient, you understand! I don't want you with her!" I feel guilty, like a cheating husband, but what the hell have I done? It'll make a funny story when it's over.

I have to remember to tell it to my father. I'll see him soon. Rikki and I have reservations to go down in February. We're spending three days in Cuernavaca with him and my stepmother, then four days alone on the beach in Puerto Vallarta. We'll certainly be ready for a vacation. This'll seem like a bad dream by then.

My father is a great storyteller but he also loves to hear a good story. I have several I'm saving for him. One involves our answering service machine.

On a recent evening, Rikki was waiting impatiently as I arrived home from work. She had gotten in a little before me and had played the messages on the machine. "There's a call I've been saving for you. You have to hear it," she said, switching on the machine.

"Rikki," began a pleasant sounding male voice, "I have feelings for you. Do you have feelings for me? If you have feelings for me, I would like to get together with you." Then the voice added, "There is no need for Robert to know about this call."

Of course, Robert, me, was listening and I immediately recognized the caller. Rikki is poor at identifying voices but she agreed with me about who it was. The incident would be perfect in a John Cheever or John Updike short story: attempted adultery on an answering service.

We thought of having a dinner party and inviting the caller, his wife, and several other couples. Toward the end of the party, we'd announce that we had something we wanted everyone to hear. "See if you can identify the mystery voice," I'd say, playing the message through our stereo. We didn't do it. We erased the tape.

My legs ache. I'm so uncomfortable. How long has it been since I saw Doria? I don't know. There are no clocks in this place. Without glasses, if there were I couldn't read the time. Besides, a curtain Doria has carelessly left partially closed, blocks any view. My secretions are building, but they're a long way from setting off the alarm. Where is Jenny? She won't help me now. Bitch Doria!

I have to move off this side. Rikki would help if she knew. Why did I let her go? I could blink my eyes and she'd understand I need help. She would try to find out what it was I wanted. She'd call Doria. She'd do something. She wouldn't have left if she'd known what would happen. She wouldn't have gone.

Charlie would help if he knew. Charlie, our only child, is a student at the University of Maryland. If he knew, he'd break in here and ask why they weren't helping me. He'd be polite—he's always polite—but he wouldn't let them ignore me. He'd demand they help.

To think of Charlie is to smile. He's everyone's favorite kid, not just mine. The best brief description of him was my father's: "He has your optimism and Rikki's enthusiasm," he'd said.

JESUS, BITCH DORIA! I have to move, don't you understand?

Charlie doesn't know. Rikki wouldn't tell him. She wouldn't tell anyone, not yet anyway. We're both like that. We have many friends but we seldom open up with any of them. Maybe we're so close that we don't need anyone else. We've always been open with Charlie, but why worry him now before we know how bad things are? Why worry anyone?

I'm drowning again, Goddamnit! The alarm is going to go off. It's so hard to breathe. Can you actually drown this way? I don't know. No, you can't, they wouldn't make a respirator that would let that happen. You're so naive. You're an asshole, a real asshole. They've knowingly built cars like the Ford Pinto with deadly design defects. So why wouldn't they build hospital machines with fatal flaws? I don't like to think this way. I could die? I could die! I don't believe that— not really. But why doesn't the alarm sound? How the fuck should I know. Oh, it's so hard to breathe.

Who's this? "You're really juicy, aren't you darling?" I blink a yes. The nurse is older than most, heavier. She suctions me quickly. Now turn me, please. No reaction. I demand you turn me! "There, that's better," she says, gathering all the disposable suctioning junk. Turn me! Please, get me off my side. I'm blinking as hard as I can. She doesn't notice. She's away, off into the gloom.

First I brood, and then I console myself. After all, there have been some net gains. I no longer need suctioning and she's pushed back the curtain. Although I can see, there isn't much to see: some other beds, the nursing station lights and the occasional ghostly figure of a nurse, moving quietly, almost floating. As each passes, I strain to see if it is Doria.

Can this really be happening? I have a profound sense of detachment. But this is not a Franz Kafka short story. This is not *The Metamorphosis*. This is me! This is happening! I still don't believe it.

I see bitch Doria. Turn me now and I forgive you everything. I'll love you forever. I'm blinking frantically. Don't you see me bitch, cunt; don't you notice? "You don't need suctioning," she says. Brilliant fucking observation, brilliant! Now turn me, bitch! "I'll be back in a short while to turn you, darling," she says, moving silently away. There is hope now. She knows I'm here and she'll be back soon.

What time is it? I haven't slept. I'm not the least bit sleepy. How can you sleep when you're so uncomfortable? Uncomfortable, hell, I'm in pain. This is all so unreasonable. No one's ever told me anything about this kind of hospital experience. All the complaints I ever heard about nurses have been somewhat humorous. I never heard a story about a horrible nurse like Doria. People don't remember the terrible things that happen to them.

Where the fuck is Doria? Has she already left for India?

Do I have a better memory for bad experiences than others do? Maybe I do. In 1955, after graduating from high school, I joined the Air Force. It was only a couple of years after the end of the Korean War where Air Force took some heavy ground casualties. The generals said those losses occurred because airmen weren't given any combat training.

They were determined not to repeat that mistake with us. Our training was brutal. Everyone said the Air Force was trying to make it tougher for us than Parris Island Marines had it. As far as I'm concerned, they succeeded. I remember them telling us that no matter how unhappy we were then, we'd remember all we were going through fondly.

As they were saying it, I knew that I would never forget the raw fear, the humiliation and the bone weariness of that terrible hot summer. I wouldn't let sentimentality cheat me out of a real memory, no matter how awful. But they were right: most men remember basic as if it were a hilarious fraternity party. When I was there, I didn't see anyone having fun.

Within months after I finished my training, the Air Force forgot the lessons of Korea and returned to its old, sloppy ways. It cut basic training down from 12 to six weeks and relaxed the discipline. So it is with the military mind.

Just as I remember basic, I will remember this night. Doria, I will remember you forever, you bitch. There is someone here. It's Doria! She didn't forget! She came back! Oh, God, she's turning me. Oh, ecstasy! I love you, Doria. I'm drowning again but you'll save me. That's it, baby. Suction, suction! Better now. Sensors are yanked away. Alarms sound. Another nurse is helping Doria replace the sensors. Now I'm sweating—terrible sweats. Swimming. They change my gown. They're filling me again with white stuff through the nose tube. I prefer ham and eggs with home fries, please.

Sweet Jesus! I hear Rikki! Could the night be over? They're turning more lights on. The night is over!

I can't see her yet, but she's arrived. I hear her. She's thanking Doria. As soon as I can talk I'll tell Rikki how awful it was. How I was ignored. "Your husband is a nice man. When I come back next month, I'll take care of him again." Never!

"That's very nice of you," Rikki says, "but by then he'll be back home. He won't need a nurse."

"I hope he's better," says Doria, "but I think he'll still be here." Fuck you, bitch! What the hell do you know? Are you a doctor?

Ralph's friend was in the hospital three months. Don't think of him.

~

Rikki looks tired but she's put makeup on for me. I love her so. "It was very lonely in the house without you," she says. "It was worse than when you are away on a trip. I was too tired to walk Ruffy. I just let him out the back. He misses you too."

"Move your leg," she asks suddenly. I try, but nothing happens. "You could do it last night. Really try," she pleads. It's no use. I blink my eyes to show her I can't.

"Blink your eyes," she says. I blink again. "Blink them now." I'm blinking them as much as I can. Can't she see that? "You're not blinking! You're just rolling them back in your head." She leans close to show me. She tries to roll her eyes back so that her pupils disappear. It makes her look frightening. Is that how I look now? Jesus!

Dr. Long is here and Rikki is telling him about my leg and my eyes. "There is no way to communicate," she says in a voice edged in panic.

"Bob," he asks, "can you move your eyes to the left and right." I can do it. It's all I have left—my eyes are the only part of me that moves. Left—right—left—right. "Good. From now on, eyes to the right means 'yes,' eyes to the left means 'no.' Got that?" I move my eyes smartly to the right. Basic training is finally paying off. That's where I learned my left from my right.

"Ask him something," Dr. Long commands.

"Do you love me?" asks Rikki. I move my eyes to the right twice. "Does that mean you love me a lot?" she asks, her face breaking into a smile for the first time today. I shift my eyes to the right once more. After teaching figure skating for some 20 years, Rikki has no trouble telling left from right.

I walked in here only 24-hours ago and it's amazing all I've learned. I now know how to breathe on a respirator—I know about catheters and tubes and nurses. I know trying to move anything but my eyes is now as futile as trying to fly by spreading my arms and jumping in the air.

If I try to move, not a muscle flickers. Nothing happens. The insulation is gone. The circuits are out. It is as impossible to move an arm as it is to move an object across a room by looking at it. I just I can't do it.

They're here for chest x-rays. Rikki and Dr. Long step out. I have a new daytime nurse. She's an attractive blonde, named Candy. She's in her late twenties—an ex-cheerleader gone hard. Like many attractive people, she has an overabundance of self-confidence.

The x-ray guy is much more interested in Candy's body than he is in mine. He must put a large film plate behind my back. Candy rolls me first one way, then the other, while this asshole jams the cold plate behind me. Because it's sticking to my skin, it hurts like hell! Now the son-of-a-bitch is shoving me around on the plate as if I'm a piece of raw liver.

While he's trying to get me in the right position, he's asking Candy about her vacation. Seems Candy just returned from Switzerland.

It feels as though he's ripping the skin on my back. I want him to stop. I'm in a panic, quickly shifting my eyes back and forth to get their attention, but they don't notice. Finally, the plate is where this asshole wants it, which feels like the most uncomfortable place he could find. He uses a light in the machine to line up the shot. The plate's so hard. Hurry please hurry!

"Don't move," he says as he steps away. I don't think he's trying to be funny.

I'm sweating again. Without warning and for no reason that I can understand, I break out in the most profuse perspiration. I'm suddenly just drenched. My gown is soaked and so are the sheets. No fever, no reason.

"What's wrong with this guy?" asks the technician as he comes to retrieve the plate. "He's soaking wet. Jeez, this is gross!" He's pulling the plate out and now it slides easily, lubricated by my perspiration.

"The sweating is normal for people with neurological conditions," Candy tells him. Nice to know I'm normal.

Rikki must wait while Candy bathes me and changes my gown and sheets. The bath is wonderful. Having someone move my body now gives me the same kind of relief you feel when you step out of a car after an all-day drive.

There is no privacy here. As Candy dries my naked body the x-ray guy bursts through the curtain. "Pictures didn't come out," he says.

Dr. Fields pushes through my curtains. "Where are my x-rays?" he demands.

"You'll have them in a little while. I have to shoot them again"

"What the hell is wrong with you people? I ordered them last night and I still don't have them."

"I don't know about last night. All I know is when I got here this morning they said get a chest on this guy. That's what I've been trying to do."

"I need those x-rays," Dr. Fields says, listening to my chest with a stethoscope.

"What a ball buster," mutters the technician after Dr. Fields is safely gone. It isn't any easier being positioned on the plate the second time than it was the first. Please make this picture good.

Rikki is finally at my bedside. As she talks, she holds my hand. "Dr. Fields thinks you probably have pneumonia. He says it's nothing to worry about, that it was almost inevitable that you'd get it after you went on the respirator." I shift my eyes to the right to show I understand. I'm not alarmed. What's a little pneumonia on top of everything else?

Dr. Schwartz, dressed in another beautiful suit, has come to test my reflexes. As Rikki watches, I feel the sharp knock of his little hammer. This time my legs and arms don't move at all. It's spooky.

"Just as I expected—he's lost his reflexes," says Dr. Schwartz.

"Is this as bad as Bob will get?" asks Rikki.

"There's no way to know," he tells her. "He'll reach a plateau and stay there before things start to reverse themselves. It'll be hard to know when that occurs."

Could my heart become paralyzed, I wonder. What else can go wrong? I am not afraid because I still feel that this isn't happening to me.

"Could, could his heart stop?" asks Rikki. Good girl!

"That's not likely. It's a different set of nerves. But that's why we have the monitors on his chest. We're watching this carefully." Then what will they do if it stops, I wonder. They can't jam an artificial heart into me to keep me alive. I know that.

"Bob," says Dr. Schwartz, "Dr. Long tells me you have trouble closing your eyes. Try to close them for me." I try. He wants an eye specialist to examine me.

"Are you having trouble seeing?" Dr. Long asks. I shift my eyes to the left to say no, even though I am. I don't have my glasses so everything is blurred.

"Do you want your glasses?" asks Rikki. "I have them in my bag." How thoughtful of her, but no thanks. I wear bifocals and if you try to use them when you're lying down, they don't work well. You're always looking through the wrong lens. What I'd like are my old, non-bifocal glasses. I have several pairs in a drawer at home, but how can I get it across that I want those and not the bifocals? I can't.

Suddenly, I need suctioning. Candy takes care of it quickly and efficiently and then turns me. Paradise on earth!

Dr. Fields has now read the x-rays. From those, and tests that show my blood has a low level of oxygen, he's confirmed that I have a very serious case of pneumonia. To fight it, they'll be giving me an antibiotic through the IV tube that's already in place in my arm. And, oh yes, they'd like to do a bronchoscopy, a suctioning of my lungs. Nothing to worry about, he assures me. Inside my body there's a huge battle being fought, but I'm not alarmed. It isn't really happening to me.

"I told Texaco that you wouldn't be in today," says Rikki. "I didn't mention the hospital." I move my eyes to the right, signaling my approval. I don't want anyone there to know what's happened. "I wanted to talk to Warren but he was in a meeting. I talked with some girl, a secretary. She took the message without asking any questions.

"I've also called the rink to say you're sick. I asked them to tell my students that I'm canceling lessons and that I won't make the competition this weekend." My eyes shift repeatedly to the left. I don't want her to start changing her life for this.

"You don't want me to cancel my lessons?" Yes, I signal. "Bob, you can't expect me to come here and also go to the rink!" she says angrily. Does she think I'm going to be here forever? "Even if you're home by this weekend," she adds, "you'll be weak and you'll need me to take care of you." I'm relieved that she doesn't think this will last very long.

The eye specialist orders them to give me drops every few hours. He's concerned that my corneas may dry out because I'm not blinking. When you blink, he explains, your eyelids moisten your eyes. Hey, you learn something everyday, even when you're paralyzed.

They don't call it intensive care for nothing. The eye drops are just another item to add to the constantly growing list of things they're doing for me. Regularly, I'm turned, washed. They feed me medicines and vitamins through the nose tube. The IV drips other medication and fluids into my arm.

An army of people are now concerned with my body. There's a never-ending troop of technicians tending the respirator. Doctors, nurses and various electronic devices constantly watch my body for any new problems.

I am amazed by how much they demand from the hospital's lab. Blood, urine and God knows what else are analyzed immediately after the doctor orders it. They take X-rays around the clock. And this is a fairly small hospital.

Overnight, I've become an industry. Think of the cost. Screw the cost! I haven't been working for one of America's largest corporations and paying for the most expensive medical insurance options all these years for nothing. Whatever it costs, it costs.

A window looks onto my bed from another ICU room. Most of the time a curtain covers it, but occasionally I notice people there staring in at me. They're visitors, not hospital employees. Who the hell are they?

Rikki sees me watching a man at the window. "I think that's the father of the boy next door," she says. "I feel so sorry for them." She's learned the son is about the age of our boy, Charlie. He had a motorcycle accident.

"The nurses say he's paralyzed for life. He'll never walk again. He's very depressed. His friends visit but he won't talk with anyone except his father. Isn't that awful?" she asks. I shift my eyes to the right twice, to show I very much agree. I couldn't bear that happening to Charlie. I'm glad I'm the one going through this and not Charlie or Rikki. I know I can take it.

Dr. Schwartz is back. He pushes the blunt end of a pin, then the sharp point against my legs and arms. I feel the difference. I have not lost my sense of touch.

Oh, Jesus! He's asking Rikki's permission to do another spinal tap. "That's Bob's decision, not mine," she says. "Ask him." He turns towards me. No, I want to scream. I never want another.

"It's very important," he says, sensing my reluctance. "We need to be certain it's Guillain-Barré you have."

Two spinal taps in two days! I remember the awfulness of the first one. I don't want it a second time. It's not fair. It's my spine. If it was his, would he let someone do it to him? But how can I say no? I'm trapped. If he says it's important, I have no choice. He's the doctor. He has all the information about how necessary the test really is. I have none. I shift my eyes to the right, giving my consent.

Rikki has much to do at home. She'll return later. I know the world goes on. Rikki, I love you.

I sense that the nurses are afraid of the doctors. I can see that Candy is and she's a fireball, aces, a model of efficiency and attractiveness. If she's afraid, they're all afraid.

"I want you to sit him up on the side of the bed," Dr. Schwartz tells her.

"I can't do that by myself. I need help."

"Well, get help," he says, angrily. Candy's right. It's impossible for her to hold me, a 190-pound pile of jelly, in a sitting position.

She leaves me to get help but she's back very soon. "Everyone is busy right now," she reports.

"Page me when things are organized," he says, stalking off.

"If only he could have waited a couple of minutes," she says. I shift my eyes to the right, in sympathy. Although I feel sorry for her, I don't like her. She pushes me around the bed as though I'm a sack of potatoes. She puts my hands in unnatural, funny-looking positions, and then mimics me. She says, "Slurp, slurp," when she suctions me.

She's knows that I'm conscious and she talks to me and that's good. But her main interest is not me but being seen as the cutest and the brightest. That negates all the good points she has as a nurse. I've learned she'll be my regular daytime nurse in the ICU.

Another nurse is now free to help her. They page Dr. Schwartz. "Dr. Schwartz, call ICU, Dr. Schwartz, call ICU." The message has a dramatic intensity. It's eerie to know it's for me. Dr. Schwartz doesn't respond. The other nurse wanders off.

Now Dr. Fields is here and he wants to do the suctioning of my lungs. "It's vital we do it now." he says, "Your lungs are filling up. You're drowning in your own secretions. Don't worry about the pain." That scares me. Pain? What pain? It hadn't occurred to me there would be pain. "We'll give you morphine."

My mind races with questions. Why morphine? Is what he's going to do that terrible? What's morphine like? I've never had an opiate. Patients become addicts in hospitals. But I've also read that doctors sometimes refuse terminally ill cancer patients morphine because they don't want them to become addicted. Is this truth or black humor? If it's true, why am I getting it now? I've also heard that morphine doesn't relieve pain; it makes you not give a damn? Is that so?

"Bob, we'll need your consent for the bronchoscopy."

Do I have a choice? It sounds like if I say no I'll die. I shift my eyes to the right. "So, it's okay with you? he asks. Again, eyes right. "Good."

"Where do you want me to put the machine?" asks Candy.

"The right side of the bed," he tells her. "I'll be back when you have it ready."

They wheel in the bronchoscopy machine and start setting it up. It looks like an antique. I hope the bronchoscopy will help reduce the need for them to suction me so often.

They've started injections of a drug called Heparin to prevent blood clots. "It's to go in the fatty part of the stomach. There's no problem with you in that department," Candy says, grabbing a handful of flab on my belly and sticking it with a needle. Ha, Ha! Fuck you, Candy!

More sweats, more baths, more suctioning, more alarms, more noise. The afternoon is passing. Candy has been to lunch. I've learned that each ICU nurse has two patients. Candy hasn't spent much time today with her other patient.

This is a good time for me to be sick, if there ever is such a time. I should be out of here and home for Christmas, ready to go on vacation to Mexico in February. I've finished putting together the next issue of the magazine and I don't owe any stories. That's because I took this last trip as a photographer, not as a writer. When you return from a long assignment as a writer, all you have are notes. It can take weeks, sometimes even months, to turn the notes into magazine pieces. A photographer returns with pictures and his job is done.

Warren and I had long hoped to take an overseas trip together, with him going as the writer and me as the photographer. When we proposed I go as the photographer this time, our bosses, who knew I had handled some photo assignments competently, saw an opportunity to save by not hiring a pricy freelancer.

We flew off as the World Series was starting in October. We worked hard, making stops in Hong Kong, Singapore, Sumatra, Sydney and New Delhi. Many of the flights were brutally long, but totally worth it. It was my first trip to the Far East. On our way home, we met our wives in Paris for a week's vacation.

When you tell people you edit a magazine for a big company, they assume it's one of those badly printed house organs with bowling scores. The Star isn't anything like that. A witty friend called it an oil slick. Our stories are not necessarily about oil but always have a Texaco angle. If we write about a small college in Kentucky, you can bet Texaco gives money to that school.

I am happy in my work. The pay is good and the hours regular, but the job lacks prestige. I do miss that special status I once had as a newspaperman. People are more interested in a junior writer from Business Week than they are in us even though we may have just returned from covering a story in Africa.

Dr. Schwartz is back to do the spinal tap. He offers no apology to Candy or me for taking so long. In fact, he doesn't talk to me at all. He's an arrogant prick. Does he know I'm still here, still me?

"I want you to sit him up on the side of the bed and hold him there," he tells Candy who has found another nurse to help her. I feel them slip my feet, then my legs over the side of the bed. They struggle to sit me up and hold me upright. I'm a huge, quivering pile of Jell-O. No nurse could do this alone. My head snaps down as I pitch forward. Mucus pours from my nose and mouth. Please hold me, please! Don't let me crash to the floor! I can't raise a hand to break the fall. The tube from the respirator pulls at my mouth; the catheter pulls my dick. Sensors pop off my chest and alarms sound.

"Turn those damn things off!" orders Dr. Schwartz. I can only look down. I don't understand why it hurts so much to sit up. Hurry, please! He jabs my back with a needle. It's the Novocain. Now we wait for it to work. My hospital gown has slipped. I stare at my stomach, bulging from lack of muscle support. For the first time, I see the catheter in my own penis. Nothing looks like me.

"Now bend him forward," Dr. Schwartz orders. He pushes against my backbone, trying to find a space between the vertebrae for his needle. I remember the sickening feeling of yesterday's spinal. What will happen if I throw up?

"Bend him more, bend him!" He shoves the back of my neck hard to push me over. My body yields slightly, and then bobs up. He tries again and again but he can't bend me enough to slip the needle in.

He stands in front of me. I see the gleaming gold bars on his Italian loafers. Real gold? "This is why he can't bend more," he says, grabbing some of my belly flab. "If he were only ten pounds less," he tells the nurses. I sense his frustration and rage. It makes me happy. I hate the bastard.

He leaves in disgust. How important was the spinal tap? Was it just something else to put on the bill? I'll never know. The nurses lay me back on the bed. Candy bathes me. She offers no solace. She says nothing. I don't care. It is enough to feel the warmth of the wet washcloth, to be lying down.

Now it's Dr. Fields turn. He's ready for the bronchoscopy. "I told you I wanted the machine on the left side," he snarls at Candy.

"No, you said the right." She's correct. I remember what he said.

"Don't tell me I'm wrong!" he shouts, storming off.

"Didn't he say the right side?" Candy asks, close to tears. I shift my eyes to the right.

A lawyer friend always insisted that all professional people are crazy. He argued that the pressures on doctors and lawyers are so great that it is impossible for them to remain sane. It's an interesting theory that became fascinating to me after he suffered a nervous breakdown. He ended up in a mental hospital where he died. The Drs. Schwartz and Fields fit his theory. They are nuts. They have to be.

Candy has shifted the machine to the left side of the bed and has Dr. Fields paged. There's no response. We wait. I stare at the ceiling. Even without my glasses, I see that the little holes in the acoustical tile are mostly paint filled. No wonder this tomb is so noisy.

Dr. Fields has returned. I half expect him to tell Candy to shift the machine to the other side but he doesn't. He explains to me that he is going to push this long plumber's snake looking instrument down through the respirator tube in my mouth and into my lungs. The snake has a light on its end that allows him to see the stuff he's going to suck out. That's the way I understand it, anyway.

He pats my shoulder reassuringly and tells me that they will be giving me morphine before the procedure. He wants me to be a brave little soldier but I'm scared. Fuck, shit, I'm scared! Dr. Field is trying to comfort me but he's not.

I have a bunch of questions but I can't ask any of them. First question, Doctor, please: Are you giving me the morphine because the procedure is incredibly painful? If this is going to hurt, how much is it going to hurt and for how long? What happens if you poke a hole in one of my lungs?

I feel the sudden stab of a needle in my right arm. It's the morphine. A warmth immediately envelopes me and fills my every cell. Hot dog! It's as though I've swallowed a great slug of whiskey, but the warmth doesn't radiate from the stomach as it does with whiskey. With this stuff, it's everywhere at once.

Now he's pushing the snake down through my mouth. I feel like a sword swallower. "Ladies and gentlemen, may I direct your attention to the center ring." It hurts, maybe not actually hurts, but it's incredibly uncomfortable.

"Give him a hundred percent oxygen," I hear Dr. Fields say. The oxygen comes through the respirator and clears my head. If the purpose of the morphine is to dull my senses, the oxygen makes them sharper.

Dr. Fields is on a high. Man, this is heaven for him. The crap in my lungs is freaking him out. "You should see this, you should see it!" He's as excited as a German U-boat commander spotting a convoy of slow-moving tankers in the North Atlantic. "Some of this stuff is like wax!" Yippee!

The machine is making terrible sucking sounds. "It's stuck," Dr. Fields tells Candy. "Turn up the power." I hear the pump rev up, then down and up again. I feel the change deep in my chest, or at least I think I do. I have an image of a car stuck in the snow, the driver gunning the engine and spinning the tires. Suddenly, the tires grab and the car lurches free.

"Look at this junk we're getting!" Dr. Fields shouts with excitement. A jar on the machines is filling with thick, yellow fluid. "This is fantastic, really fantastic," he coos. Peering through his instrument, he's on the same high as a fashion photographer during a big shoot. He's seeing things no one else can see, but instead of some babe's cleavage, it's some horrible crud in my lungs.

When I'm working as a photographer I sometimes have an overwhelming urge to show someone else what I see in the viewfinder. Dr. Fields has the same urge. "Here look," he says, handing the instrument to Candy. She peers into it, but she doesn't share his enthusiasm.

"Very interesting," she says.

The bronchoscopy goes on and on. I use an old dentist chair trick of mine, thinking of other things. This is for my own good and when it's over, it's over, I tell myself. Dr. Fields must pause often so Candy can suction me. Maybe I'll need less suctioning now.

Dr. Fields' face is flush with excitement. Maybe he's near the end. "I'm almost done with that lung," he mutters. Oh, no, this is going to go on forever. If I had only one lung, like a cousin of mine who lost one to cancer, I'd be finished now, I think.

I haven't smoked for three months. I'm damn proud of that. I finished the trip around the world without a cigarette. Warren, who somehow manages to smoke only a couple of cigarettes a day, didn't think I'd make it. I am so glad I did. Imagine lying here with everything going on and dying for a cigarette.

The car is stuck in the snow again. "There's more down there but I'm not going to be able to get it," Dr. Fields says. He sounds tired, exhausted. "Tomorrow is another day," he adds brightly. "We'll x-ray and do another bronchoscopy."

Holy shit! I thought you only got one of these a lifetime. "Okay with you, Bob?" I shift my eyes twice to the left. No! Fuck no! You can get your jollies some other way, you fucking maniac.

"Bob, be reasonable. If your lungs are filled again, we have to do the bronchoscopy. Otherwise, you'll drown. You'll die! You understand that, don't you?" It is a question with only one answer. My eyes slide to the right.

"I'll try and avoid a bronchoscopy," he promises. "I know they're no fun." My eyes don't move. Bronchoscopies are no fun for me but they seem better than sex for him. "We'll see what happens tomorrow," he says. I stare straight, moving my eyes neither to the left nor to the right.

Rikki is back. She's holding my hand. No doctors are around. The day shift nurses are leaving. The night shift is coming on. "I'll bet you'll miss Doria," says Rikki. I shift my eyes to the right. We are usually so honest with each other, but this is beyond my abilities to explain. It doesn't matter anyway. Doria is on her way to India.

"I know the head nurse," Rikki tells me. "She took skating lessons from me years ago. I told her you wanted a nurse just like Doria." I can hardly believe that she's saying this. Why the fuck doesn't she let things be!

"I want you to have only the best care," she says with a sudden sob. "I want the best nurses, the best doctors— everything." I move my eyes to the right again and again. I want to comfort her. She couldn't know about Doria. How could she. It must be so hard for her.

"Do you want me to call your parents?" I shift my eyes to the left twice. It would be crushing for them, especially my father. He's buried a wife and he's buried a daughter. That's tragedy enough for one life. He's 79 and frail. He can't do anything for me—nothing at all.

"Is there anyone I should tell?" My eyes go to the left. If no one knows, it will go away. It is our secret, my darling.

The terrible sweats have returned. I'm dripping wet, my gown and the sheets are soaked. It is not unusual to me, but it's the first time Rikki has seen it. She calls the new night nurse, a dark-haired, heavyset woman in her forties named Helen. Rikki is alarmed, but Helen treats it all calmly.

Helen is going to bathe me and change my sheets. It will take a while so Rikki will have to wait outside the curtains of my cubicle.

"Do you want me to wait?" she asks. I shift my eyes quickly to the left, telling her no. I know her so well. The fact that she even asks, says she wants to leave. And I want her to go because as soon as she leaves the nurse will turn me off my side. And during the bath and changing of the sheets, she'll turn me again and again. Go, I want you to go.

Rikki tenderly strokes my face. I feel my beard. I haven't shaved in over 24-hours.

"Oh darling, I don't like this. I want you home." She bends and kisses me. "You love me. I know you love me." My eyes shift twice to the right. Just go. "I'll be back first thing in the morning," she promises, and then she's off.

Rikki has been gone a long time now and there's no sign of Helen. Where the fuck is she? The sweat is drying on my body. What's wrong with these nurses? This is fucking outrageous. I've been here on this side for how long? I don't know and I don't care. I want to move; I have to move!

Damn, I forgot to tell Rikki about them trying to do a spinal tap or the bronchoscopy. I didn't tell her about the morphine, or Doria or Candy or the doctors. Of course you didn't, you asshole! You can't talk—you can't tell anyone anything. I keep forgetting.

What a remarkable experience to live through. I'd be frightened if it was forever but it is not forever. I'll make a full recovery. I'll be better soon.

Where the hell is that nurse? Did she die?

I've always been an incredible optimist. There's a story about four year-old twin brothers who wake up Christmas morning and rush into the living room to open their presents. Under the tree is an enormous pile of manure. "All Santa left is a bunch of horse shit!" the first twin sobs.

"Oh, great!" shouts his brother. "There has to be a pony somewhere."

I'm the second brother. I've always believed there's a pony behind every pile of horseshit. The glass isn't half-empty; it's half-full, and so on.

My sister, Joan, was the opposite. To her, horseshit was horseshit, and the glass was always half empty.

My optimism was part of what made me my father's favorite. He was unfair to my sister. I realized that even when I was very young. Of course, I sometimes took advantage of the situation, but I tried not to. I thought Joan was so down because he so often picked on her.

By the age of nine or ten, I started telling him I thought he was unfair to her. He's often disarmingly honest so he didn't deny it. "Joan was a pain in the ass from the day she was born," he'd say, as if that justified his behavior.

After I learned how environment can influence a person's life, I told him that I thought he'd shaped her temperament. "No, Bobby, Joan was always that way." I doubted that could be true.

He loved her but she constantly annoyed him. The more she tried, the worse it got. It was painful to watch. When she got older, she knew he disapproved of the men in her life even though he never said it. How could they have pleased him? None were writers or even read enough to win him over. One did have the wit, however, to call him a liberal Archie Bunker. The description amused him because he knew it was on the mark.

When Charlie was born and I started learning firsthand about kids, I began to think that maybe my father had a point about my sister's personality. Charlie was cheerful from the start. As we got to know other infants, we realized that they also seemed to have been born with temperaments. We watched some of these kids grow up, saw *many of them go through trying times, yet their personalities seemed unchanged.*

I realize that to a scientist this is all evidence of nothing. Where was my control? How big was my sample? These arguments are not for me. I know what I know. I can't spend a lifetime in studies. I believe a person's basic personality is encoded before he's born and, short of the most severe physical or psychological trauma, it remains basically unchanged to the end.

Relaxing over a beer on a beach in Mexico a couple of years ago, I told my father that I finally agreed with him about Joan. She probably had been annoying to him from the day she was born.

He wasn't the least bit surprised to hear that I'd come around to his way of thinking. "So if the way she was wasn't her fault," I asked, "why did you pick on her for it?" The question was moot. By then Joan had been dead for several years.

"Bobby, I couldn't help it," my old man said, looking morose.

So please don't credit me for being an optimist, or blame my sister for the way she was. I am not morose. I am generally cheerful. I always have been and I believe that no matter what happens I always will be. It is not a matter of free will. I do not deserve credit for my temperament anymore than Joanie deserved blame for hers.

Helen! Where is that fucking nurse? Bitch! Cunt! Sticks and stones will break her bones but names will never hurt her. I can't throw sticks or stones; I can't even call her names.

My back aches where it presses against the pillow that is propping me up. It feels like it is made of cement. I know it isn't. It's just that I have been lying here so long.

My secretions are building and they'll help attract attention. Eventually, they'll get so bad that they'll cause the big alarm on the respirator to honk. I've learned the alarm sounds when there's too much backpressure. This should never happen. They should fire a nurse for neglect every time it sounds. The idea comforts me.

Helen is finally here but I've waited so long that the sweat has dried on my body. I want to scream at her. She acts as though everything is okay. I don't want her to suction me. I don't want her to bathe me. Just turn me, bitch. Get me off this side. That's all I need.

Is there no way to speed this woman? She suctions. She gets the towels. She gets the soap. She gets the basin of water. Finally, she pulls the pillow from behind me and I roll on my back. Relief! The relief!

The bath has been over for a long time. The intensive care unit has settled into its nighttime still. An occasional series of kerplunks come from the nursing station. Sometimes there's an isolated kerplunk. What is that noise? I know I know it.

My respirator gives me a deep breath at regular intervals. I try to count the number of ordinary breaths before the big one. I can't concentrate that long. I hear a television set in the distance talking about Poland. Trouble there? I don't give a damn.

It's nice to lie here without an urgent need. I don't need to be suctioned; I don't need to be turned. What would I ask for if Helen appeared and I could speak? I'm not thirsty or hungry. They keep me filled with white stuff. Jesus, I hope they don't overfeed me. I don't want to be the first man in history to gain weight in the ICU.

Helen is back. No alarms, nothing, she simply appears on her own. She suctions me. She's not great but I have to admit she's better than Doria. "Your wife is very pretty," she says. I shift my eyes once to the right in agreement.

She's gone without turning me. I wish she'd turned me. God, do I! I'm not in any pain, nothing aches, but to be rolled over in bed is pure pleasure. I wish they'd do it every twenty minutes. That's all I ask of life now.

Alarms sound, nurses quietly pass, and there is the kerplunk. No sign of Jenny, the nurse I love. Is she off? I listen to my respirator. I doubt if I could breathe without it. Funny, how I no longer hear it unless I try to. Guess it's what they mean by white noise. They're staring at me from the paralyzed boy's window. Screw them. I must look strange.

What time it is now? It has to be very late. Helen has been back twice to suction me. She's much better than Doria. No sleep for me. I haven't slept since I've been here. How very odd.

I've had the terrible sweats. Helen is finishing my bath and is again ready to change the sheets. "Your fat is different from my fat," she says quietly. Yeah, I think, you have a lot more of it. You got fat eating steaks and good food. I got fat eating junk. "I'm not beautiful like your wife. I'm not." I can't argue with that.

"You're a writer. You know what my husband is?" I haven't a clue. "He's a transit cop. A transit cop in New York City," she whines. "Some people are people of quality and some people aren't. You and your wife are; me and my husband aren't." She finishes changing the bed in silence. Doctors aren't the only crazy ones in this hospital.

Morning has come. I recognize the signs. The lights are going on. The pace is picking up. "Hey, honey, get me a *Daily News*," cries a very New York City voice. I can't see him but I've heard the voice before. He's been telling everyone who'll listen that he had a heart attack while driving on the Thruway.

He has to wait for the paper, a nurse informs him, because the gift shop hasn't yet opened.

"Then help me go to the bathroom. I got to go bad."

"I'll bring you a bed pan," says the nurse. "You're not allowed out of bed."

"I'm sixty one years old. I ain't ever used a bedpan. I ain't ever been sick."

"There's a first time for everything," she replies. She's right. Being healthy all your life means nothing. That was then, this is now. It's now that counts.

Rikki is here. She's soft and tender, filled with love. She kisses me and holds me as best she can without disturbing my tubes and wires. She has made a sign to go on the wall behind my bed "Bob can talk" it says. "Ask him a question. He moves his eyes to the right to say yes, to the left to say no." She's drawn a cartoon of two shifty eyes on it.

"I want them to know that you're still a person, that they can talk to you and that you can understand. Is it all right to put it up?" I move my eyes to the right. Sure it's all right. Only you could have thought of this.

"Bob" she says, holding my hand. "Max called this morning to invite us out to dinner with him and Phyllis. I told him you're in the hospital. I'm sorry but I just broke down and told him." Oh, shit, why did you have to go and do that!

"He is so upset. He wanted to do something so I asked him to find any articles he could about Guillain-Barré and get them for me." I know Max will be good at that. He's a guidance counselor across the street at Nyack High School. He's done graduate work and knows how to research things. Max is a fantastic friend. Ask him a favor and it's done. Don't think twice. He just does it. Period.

"While I was talking to Max, I decided to call Alan Zimmerman and ask him to find out who's the best doctor in New York City for Guillain-Barré. I want to talk to the best expert we can find." I shift my eyes in approval. Rikki, baby, you're cooking.

Alan is one of our oldest friends. We all met in 1960 during my early newspaper career on the White Plains newspaper.

Alan and I were reporters, and Rikki was the editor's secretary. Alan dated Rikki a few times before she and I became serious.

He went on to become a writer and producer of radio and television news. A few years after Rikki and I were married, he married Josepha, a model-beautiful German woman. If there is a best doctor for Guillain-Barré, Alan will find him.

"I also told Wanda," says Rikki. Oh, Jesus, Rikki, why don't you hold a press conference? I understand telling Max and Alan. You had good reasons, but Wanda? I shift my eyes repeatedly to the left to show I'm angry.

"What could I do?" she asks, exasperated. "Wanda left a lot of messages on the answering service. She's been wondering what happened since you called her. She checked with the hospital and they told her you were in intensive care. Naturally, she was worried. I had to let her know."

I move my eyes to the right. Okay, okay. I don't blame you. I don't know what's going on. So the cat's out of the bag. We've gone public, as they say at the White House.

"I have to call Charlie soon and tell him what's happened. I don't want him hearing it from someone else. I'm going to have to tell my parents and my brother and sister for the same reason. Do you want Charlie to come home?"

Eyes left! Eyes left! No! Hell no! Tears flood my eyes. I don't want Charlie to see me this way. I don't want anyone to see me this way. Ever!

"It's all right darling, it's all right. Charlie won't come," Rikki says, wiping away my tears, and tenderly patting my hand. The tears have set off a flood of mucus. Rikki runs out to find Candy. I'm drowning again in mucus. The bronchoscopy has done nothing to cut the flow.

Candy is very good at suctioning, but being suctioned is awful. My extremities tingle and my nose tears. But I've already rationalized these discomforts. It is the price of not drowning in my own secretions. The price is high but it's worth it. And, I have no choice.

Rikki should go home for a while, Candy says. They've scheduled me for more x-rays, blood tests, a bath and a linen change—busy! busy! busy!

That was long ago. Hours have passed. How long since Rikki's been gone? I don't know. There is little sense of time here. It is like a gambling casino—no windows and no clocks. Rikki's visits are all I look forward to. I don't look forward to meals as I usually do. I'm never hungry now anyway. I don't sleep.

There's a new x-ray technician. He's as rough on me as the one I had yesterday. I make an instant judgment: the x-ray technicians here are a bunch of brutes. By contrast, the people who tend the respirator seem gentle and truly concerned. Before they make adjustments to the machine or change its hoses, they explain what they are going to do.

"Are you really six feet tall?" Candy asks as she checks my chart. Eyes right. Of course I am.

We are waiting for Dr. Fields and another bronchoscopy. Will I get more morphine? I only care because it breaks the monotony. Candy has the machine to the left of the bed, per Dr. Fields' instructions. "You don't look six feet tall. Are you sure you are?" Again, I shift my eyes right.

Candy suddenly plops down beside me. It both startles and frightens me. My body twists painfully from the added weight on the mattress. A few sensors pop off. It's all funny as hell to Candy. "Let's see," she says, stretching out and measuring her height against mine, "I'm five nine. Yeah, I guess you're six feet."

She's up laughing, putting the sensors back. I feel humiliated. I hate you, you, unprofessional bitch.

I hear Dr Fields. "Is everything ready?"

"Yes, Doctor, it is."

"The machine—on what side of the bed did I tell you I wanted it?" He rushes around the bed. Anger flames his gentle face. He's insane!

"The left side."

"The left side? The left side! I distinctly told you the right side."

"But remember," she pleads, "I asked you twice which side and you said the left side both times."

"Nurse, I'm not going to stand here and argue with you about this. Just move the machine."

Dr. Fields is gone. "Don't you remember him telling me the left side?" Candy asks, distraught. I lie. I shift my eyes to the left to say I don't remember. Fuck you, Candy!

Now Rikki is back. She's talked to Charlie and her parents. She says she's told them the situation in a very factual way, emphasizing that I will fully recover. "Charlie wanted to come home on the next plane, but I told him not to."

Soon, everyone will know.

Dr. Fields invades our privacy. "Hate to break this up but it's time for the bronchoscopy." He acts like a high school principal who has caught the cute couple necking in the hall. He seems dopey but normal, not like the madman I know he is.

Rikki kisses me goodbye. She'll be back later. I know she feels safe, leaving me with Dr. Fields, but she hasn't seen him operating his machine.

It's just us three behind the curtain—Dr. Fields, Candy and me. Morphine time! Set 'em up, Joe. Time to get high! Hit me again, Daddy. What's this? He's getting right down to business. No shots. He already has the fucking tube down my throat. "Look at this stuff," he says. "It's worse than yesterday."

He sounds petulant, like a housewife who has vacuumed and "now just look at this mess!" Stamp your little foot, Dr. Fields. Full speed ahead! "Hundred percent oxygen!" he orders. At least he's not forgotten that, but I'm pissed. I'm not getting my morphine. You'd think I'm big on drugs. Not so. Wrong generation. The only drug I ever tried is marijuana, and I haven't had any of that in a long while.

There was a time when every suburban party had a group in a corner smoking a joint. No more. I think most of my generation likes booze better. I certainly do. Pot makes me introverted, less social. Booze lets me at least feel I'm having a good time.

"Why do you drink so much, Sir Winston?" the young reporter asks the great man.

"I drink to get rid of the warts."

"But sir, you have no warts."

"Not my warts, you fool," roars Churchill, "Other people's warts."

I'm sure that I don't drink as often, as much or as well as Churchill, but I drink for the same reason: after a little alcohol, everyone—both men and women—seem more attractive and more interesting.

I've never had a drinking problem, but I do eat too much and I did smoke too much. Dr. Fields doesn't need booze or marijuana. He gets high sucking lungs. Let him get high on me. I know he thinks I'll die if this doesn't work so suck on, my good doctor. Even though dying does not seem an immediate possibility to me, let me be clear: I want to live. I want to go to Mexico in February and sit again with my father in the sun. I want to see Charlie grow up. I want to get old with Rikki and become a grandfather. I want to go to the Blauhuts's party tomorrow night. I want to live. Suck on, you bastard!

The night has returned. I lie, eyes open. I do not sleep. Is this rest? They have pushed, punctured, suctioned, filled, inflated, drained, bruised, washed and manhandled my body in ways I can't recall. The beat of the respirator is constant. I'm dreadfully lonely. Is this life? I don't want to live this way. Maybe they should let me die.

~

A man screams. He's out of his head with pain and drugs. I've heard the nurses talking. They say he was driving a steamroller on the Tappan Zee Bridge when a car smashed into it, knocking him to the roadway. The steamroller kept going, crushing one of his legs. The doctors have amputated it.

I know the accident scene—the flashing red lights and the traffic backup. When we were first married and very young we lived in a tiny boathouse a quarter-mile from that bridge. The squeal of brakes, followed by the clash of metal and the delicate tinkle of broken glass often jolted us awake. In the deep silence that followed, Rikki would grab for me as we held our breath, hoping the hellish screams of people in pain wouldn't shatter the quiet, making the hair rise on the back of my neck. Many of the victims of those accidents ended up here.

"He keeps trying to pull out his tubes," I overhear a nurse saying about the steamroller driver.

"When a patient does that," another replies, "it means that the tubes are ready to come out anyway."

I want to yank out all my tubes to show that I don't need them, but I can't. My eyes can't pull tubes and my eyes are all I can move. So, I guess my tubes stay.

What will I do when I first move? That's easy. I'll roll over in bed. Turn me please, oh Nurse Helen, angel in white in the night. Where art thou, Bitch?

It's much later now. There has been much excitement and noise near the steamroller man's bed. I don't know what happened, but he's not dead—he's still yelling.

I hear my favorite nurse, Jenny. "He pushed his hand right up my dress and started pulling at my panties," she tells another nurse. Let me at him. I'll kill him, I think. But Jenny isn't angry she's titillated. I'm jealous. Beats pulling at tubes, I'd say.

Another new patient arrives. I don't see her, of course, but I hear the nurses. A drug overdose, they gossip, and she has two small children at home. "There is going to be a lot of this, now that the holiday season is starting," says Candy who has just come to work.

"Did you think of your children when you took those pills?" I hear Candy ask her. I love you most for your sensitivity, Candy.

X-ray time! The fat technician is here. Jesus, what's this bastard doing. Get Candy to help, you dumb fuck. He's trying to lift me by himself to shove the plate in, but he's not able to do it. He's hurting me. He's twisting my body and I'm losing sensors. My alarms are ringing. Candy is here. "What the hell are you trying to do?" she asks, laughing. She thinks it's funny.

"Help me shove the plate under this guy. I have to do another chest x-ray on him," he says, grabbing both my hands and yanking me toward him. My head, unsupported, snaps back and mucus spills from my mouth. My arms ache. Why is this so painful? It wouldn't have bothered me at all before.

To the technician, I'm not a human being. I can't move or talk. I am a lump of meat. Candy clears out so he can shoot his picture. The machine emits its sinister buzz. I hope the x-rays make him sterile, sparing the world more fuck-heads like him.

Is it safe for me to have this many x-rays? All I know is that x-ray damage is cumulative and you should avoid it if you can. I get two chest x-rays ever day, except when they screw up and have to repeat them. This happens surprisingly often. If I could talk, I'd ask Dr. Fields why I have to have so many. Can't he see what's in my lungs during a bronchoscopy? Isn't that enough?

The woman with the overdose is retching violently. They've given her charcoal to absorb the drugs and make her vomit. Candy is elated. "I dumped the whole mess down the sink, charcoal and all. It's amazing what the plumbing can take," she says.

"Do you use drugs?" she asks me suspiciously. Eyes left.

Rikki has arrived. Today is Saturday, December 5, my fourth day in the hospital, she announces. The doctors have warned her that I'll lose track of time unless she reminds me of the date.

She's brought in a picture to put on a wall near my bed. I know she wants to convince the people who take care of me that I am a normal person with a loving family. The 5X7 print shows all of us—Rikki sits on our backyard bench, trying to hold our squirming dog, Ruffy, on her lap. Charlie and I flank her. This is our most recent family photo. Charlie's best friend, Willie, took it with my camera. It has too much contrast, too many shadows and bright spots, but it evokes the warm spring day and a moment in our lives. When I see it, I ache for home. I miss the house, the dog, my normal life. When will this all end?

"I want Charlie to come home," Rikki says. My eyes go to the left. No! I told you I don't want him to see me like this.

"I called him late last night," she continues, ignoring me, "and we talked for maybe an hour. He so much wants to come and see you and I need him," she pleads.

Suddenly, I also want him here. It's right that he come. I love him totally. He's old enough to share this with us and he should. Rikki shouldn't be alone. I shift my eyes to the right and Rikki smiles.

"I'm so glad you changed your mind," she says, clutching my hand. "It will be so good to have him home." Eyes right again. She starts to leave to make the call, then pauses. "What I'm so afraid of," she says, "is that you'll get worse. The doctors don't know if you've reached a plateau. They just don't know. You could lose the use of your eyes and not be able to communicate at all. I don't want that to happen," she adds with an unexpected sob.

I shift my eyes to the right. I won't let it happen. I can't. "I'm going to call Charlie now," she says, wiping at her tears.

Charlie has only been back at school a short while since his Thanksgiving break. We got along well while he was here. We actually enjoyed cleaning the roof gutters together. We always save that job for Thanksgiving weekend after the last leaf has fallen. He had always helped, but this year, for the first time, he took over, and I felt as if I were the one helping. Before he returned to school, he told me I had treated him more like an equal than ever before. I guess I had. He's growing up.

"Charlie will be home tonight," Rikki says as she returns. She's beaming now and has lots of other news she hasn't had a chance to tell me. Alan Zimmerman called with information on New York doctors and hospitals. The best doctor in New York for Guillain-Barré is Dr. Nigel Ramsbotham, a neurologist at Columbia-Presbyterian Hospital. Rikki will call him first thing Monday morning.

Max came through with two articles on Guillain-Barré. "I've looked through them and they say what the doctors say: you do get better." Seeing it in print has reassured Rikki. I've had no doubts.

"My father and my brother are coming to the hospital to see me and they'd love to visit you." No! Eyes left. Not! "Is there anyone you want to have visit?" I would like to see Dale and Stanley, but it's impossible to tell her. I answer no again. "Are you sure?"

She begins naming friends. After a few, she mentions Dale. My eyes go right. She's surprised. "Anyone else?" Yes. More names, then Stanley's. Yes. Now she's puzzled. I know she wonders why, of all my friends, I ask for them.

It's because they have both survived recent life-threatening crises. Dale suffered a stroke and Stanley went through open-heart surgery. They'll be empathetic. They'll understand that it is not my fault that I'm sick. And maybe they'll know how vulnerable I feel lying on this bed.

While Candy is suctioning me, Dr. Fields talks to Rikki. I catch only part of what he's saying about lungs and x-rays and shadows. Oh Jesus, no, he's telling her I have lung cancer. Rikki looks so grave. Here's the payoff for those thousands of cigarettes I've smoked since I was sixteen. That's almost 30 years of puffing away. I quit too late. Do the crime, do the time.

The suctioning is over, but I still can't hear Rikki and Dr. Fields. They are too far away. Did he say something about my mother? He must be talking about the terrible history of cancer on my mother's side of the family. I knew someday it would get me. They're coming over now. They're going to tell me. This is when I find out how it all ends for me.

"Darling," Rikki says, "Dr. Fields has some bad news." Let me have it! "He's going to a convention tomorrow."

"You'll be in good hands, Bob," he says jovially, but I barely hear. "My associate, Dr. Nagelberg, will take care of you while I'm gone."

I don't care if you leave, you crazy, fucking bastard, but first tell me, do I have cancer? Is Nagelberg a cancer specialist? That's all I want to know.

"I have fully briefed him about your condition and, as I told your wife, I have complete faith and confidence in his abilities. If I didn't, I wouldn't practice medicine with him.

"Bob," he goes on, "I want to make you more comfortable, get that tube out of your mouth. I've explained to your wife that I'm recommending a tracheotomy. They'll make a small incision in your throat. That way the tube from the respirator can go directly there." It means they're going to take a biopsy of my throat. I knew it.

"It's really nothing to worry about. The surgeon will perform the procedure right here in your bed. The operation is quite fashionable," he adds, beaming. "Elizabeth Taylor had it."

"Do I have your permission to go ahead? It will make you a lot more comfortable." I answer yes. I want them to go after that tumor as soon as they can.

"Your x-rays show you need another bronchoscopy. I'll be back in a little while to take care of it." I shift my eyes to the right. Who cares about that now? There are worse things.

Rikki says nothing to me about cancer. They must be planning to tell me later, maybe when Dr. Nagelberg comes on the case and after Charlie is here.

It's much later. Dr. Fields has finished the bronchoscopy. I couldn't believe he could do it again, but he threw another fit about the machine being on the wrong side. It's almost funny. I've heard nothing more about cancer.

Rikki has had a meeting in a waiting room with her father, brother and sister-in-law and a bunch of our friends.

Everyone thinks we should look into moving to a New York City hospital. I shift my eyes in agreement. One of the advantages of living less than 40 minutes from the city is that its great hospitals are so close.

Stanley is waiting to see me. Rikki probably thinks that I want to see him because he's a psychologist. She leads him to my bed. I watch with detachment. Stanley seems shocked. Jesus, I must be hard to look at. Easy does it, Stan, it's not that bad.

"It's just like you to get something no one ever heard of," he says, with feigned indignation. "At least you could have come down with something that had a name your friends could pronounce. Damn inconsiderate." Not bad material, but Stan, you sure look nervous.

"The important thing for you to remember," he adds, "is that people get better from this. I checked with a physician friend of mine and that's what he said. So it's no bullshit." I shift my eyes to the right. Good man, Stanley!

Stanley is gone, but Rikki is here, back from having supper. We're anxious to see Charlie. Dale is picking him up at Newark Airport. While we wait, Rikki asks me how I feel about Candy. She saw Candy tease me several times today and guessed that I didn't like it. Do I like Candy? No. Do I want Rikki to see if she can get me another nurse? Does it bother me that much? Yes! The head nurse Rikki knows will be on in the morning. Rikki will speak to her. Maybe I'll be rid of Candy tomorrow, but what then? I'll worry later.

The boy in the next room is leaving. They are taking him by ambulance to a rehab hospital. I don't know what that means. The one-legged steamroller driver must be gone too. No one's mentioned him. If he's here, he's quiet. They've discharged the woman with the drug overdose, sent her home to her children.

Rikki tells me that she wants Marilyn, a friend who is estranged from her husband, to come and live in our house with her while I'm in the hospital. "How do you feel about that?" she asks. I feel terrible, that's how I feel. I don't want Marilyn moving in. I don't want my illness changing our lives more than it has. Why doesn't she wait until the cancer kills me? I move my eyes to the left.

There is some noise outside my partially drawn curtains. Charlie has arrived. I hear his voice. Rikki rushes out to meet him. I see Dale. His big, shaggy face is so mournful. He pats one of my hands. "Charlie's here. I picked him up at the airport," he tells me needlessly.

Dale is so somber. I must look to him as if I am going to die. I want to say, it's all right, Dale. I'm going to be okay. But maybe he knows I have cancer. No, Rikki wouldn't tell him before she told me.

"I'm going now," he says, bending to kiss me on the cheek. It is such a tender, loving thing to do. No one with a beard has ever kissed me. His whiskers prick my face. It is as though he thinks he may be seeing me alive for the last time. Oh, Dale, no, I want to say but he's gone and I cannot talk.

The smell of the fresh night air on Charlie tells me that December has finally gone cold. He is near my bed and crying. Sobs rack his shoulders. Don't cry, my big boy, don't cry. Rikki has left us alone.

"Bob," he says, "I feel so bad. This shouldn't happen to you." He kisses and hugs me as best he can, his tears wetting my face. My eyes brim with tears. I am so sorry that he has to go through this. "Oh, Bob," he moans.

He's always called us by our first names. People often assume it's some affectation of ours. The truth is more complicated. When Charlie was born, a membrane tied his tongue to the floor of his mouth. His pediatrician assured us that he'd outgrow the condition, but he didn't. When a surgeon finally snipped the membrane away, Charlie immediately began talking in complete sentences. Since he's an only child he had never heard anyone call us mom and dad. That's why he began using our first names. We'd have felt pompous correcting him.

"Are you scared?" he asks, regaining some of his composure. He watches my eyes for the answer. I say no. I'm so glad Rikki told him that I can talk with my eyes.

"Are you in any pain?" Again, I say no, but I am in pain. I am cramped and ache to be turned. I can't do anything about it until Rikki is back near my bed.

"Nothing hurts?" Nothing hurts, I lie. He seems reassured. I see him look around and spot the sign Rikki made. He's a very visual person.

"That's so neat," he says, "so Rikki." Eyes right! It is; he's correct.

"Bob, I was so anxious to see you after she told me you were in the hospital. I wanted to come right then. When the plane took off and I felt its power, I kept thinking, 'It's taking me to see my Pop.' No one had a more important reason to be on that plane than me."

My eyes shift to the right. "When Rikki called, she sounded upset but she said you were going to be all right. Then, I met Dale at the airport and I got scared. He was so quiet. I thought maybe you had died. Now that I'm here and can see you, I feel so much better." Yes. It's so good that he's here

"Is Rikki doing all right?" I shift my eyes twice to the right. She's doing great. No one could do better. "That's something, the way you've learned to do that with your eyes. You'll have the strongest eye muscles in the world when this is over." I move my eyes back and forth crazily. He's still such a kid.

"Bob, I couldn't believe the view I had of Manhattan as we flew into Newark. It's so clear out. You always told me that no matter where you've been, you look for that view when you come back. You still think that sight is one of the greatest in the world, don't you?" Eyes right.

He's relaxing. He's talking with me the way he always does, but I can only answer yes or no with my eyes. I think longer answers. "Is it hard to breathe on the machine?" No. I'm completely used to it. Its rhythm is my rhythm now. "Does the tube in the nose bother you?" No, not especially, but all the tubes bother me. I'm so fucking uncomfortable most of the time.

Jenny, my favorite nurse, passes and Charlie notices her. He looks at me with a smile that says he thinks she's a pretty girl. I wag my eyes in agreement. "All right, Bob," he says with a laugh.

They'd make a nice looking couple. Charlie is slim, close to six feet tall, with Rikki's coloring, blonde hair and blue eyes. Because of his high cheekbones, his eyes have an almost Asian cast. Maybe that's some of my mother's Russian background.

When Rikki joins us, I swing my eyes left and right to tell her something's wrong. She quickly gets Helen. Does my mouth need suctioning, they ask. No. My nose? No. Is the pillow under my head all right? Yes. They keep firing the same questions at me over and over, not asking the one question I want to hear. It's maddening. Finally, they do ask. "Do I want to be turned?" Yes! Yes! Yes!

Rikki and Charlie are gone now. They'll be back in the morning. It's so good to have him with us. Maybe I don't have cancer after all. If they thought I had it, Rikki wouldn't let this much time go by without telling me.

I know she's worried about me losing the use of my eyes. That worries me too. If that happened, it would be the end. I'd want to die. If I didn't have my eyes, I couldn't tell them when something's wrong. It's hard to imagine being totally cut off like that, but it must happen to people. Helen Keller was like that. She also was deaf. I'd hear everything, but not be able to respond. I'd be blind, dumb and paralyzed, yet my mind would be clear. I'd go insane. I know I would. I have to be able to communicate. This won't happen to me! I can't let it!

There's the kerplunk again. I hear it all the time but I'm more aware of it when things are quiet. I wish I could remember where I've heard that sound before. It looks as though I'm in for another night without sleep. Why can't I sleep? The doctors and nurses don't seem concerned. Do they even notice? No one asks if I sleep. No one seems to care. Kerplunk!

If any family can survive this thing, we can. Helen, crazy as she may be, is right about us. We are successful people. We do things well. My job is satisfying and we're happy and financially secure. We travel. We have a house we love and a solid marriage. Charlie is on his way to a career in graphic arts. Rikki's mail order business, sprung from an idea she had, is a roaring success. Most of all, we love each other.

But our life hasn't been all ice cream and cake. We started our marriage dirt poor and we've both suffered disappointments and defeats. I haven't achieved all I wanted and neither has Rikki. After the *World-Telegram and Sun* folded, I tried to get a job on *The New York Times*. They didn't hire me. For years, I dreamed of being a great novelist but the novel I wrote wasn't very good and no one was interested in publishing it. In 1960, Rikki was the fifth best woman figure skater in the United States. Only the top three go to the Olympics. There have been other setbacks, other losses, but we have survived and gone on. We will survive this. I know it. We do things well. We are successful people.

The nights here are endless. I'm always waiting, waiting to be suctioned, waiting to be bathed, but mostly waiting to be turned. When Rikki is here, things happen faster. I signal her that there's something wrong and she gets a nurse. We go through the litany of questions until they hit what I want. At night I wait.

The Blauhuts's dinner party was tonight. Sweet Jesus, what a silly thing to worry about. But I wanted Rikki to go, to carry on as though things were normal. I'm sure she didn't go. I have to remember, things aren't normal. There's no doubt of that. Still, most of the time, I feel this isn't really happening to me. How could it be?

Must be after midnight. Maybe even early in the morning. Who knows? They're here for X-rays. Not the fat technician this time, but another one. He has Helen help get me on the plate. It always hurts like hell. The plate itself is cold and hard. Hope they don't have to re-shoot it. There must be a better way.

I hear Charlie and Rikki. It doesn't seem possible that the hours have gone, but another night is over. Rikki sounds happier than she has in days. Having Charlie home always perks her up.

They peer at my eyes to see if they're still working. I swing them back and forth, to show that they are. "Try and close them," says Rikki. It feels as though I am, but the way she and Charlie stare, I know I'm still only rolling them back in my head.

They've brought a new hand-lettered poster. It's a checklist, covering suctioning, pillows, lights and turning. "With this," Charlie says, "we won't forget to ask about all the things you might need like we did yesterday." What a fantastic idea! They should be in the business of inventing aids for patients.

He holds the poster close so I can read it. "Bob, you sure you don't want your glasses?" Yes, I'm sure. "We can't understand why you don't want them, but we'll keep asking in case you change your mind. It's hard to get used to you without glasses," he adds.

"I called your parents last night." Rikki tells me. "I was afraid if I didn't, they'd find out what happened from someone else. So many people now know that you're sick. Someone might call them to ask how you are."

Tears flood my eyes. I didn't want my father to know. This must be such devastating news for him. "They took it very well," Rikki says softly. "They asked how to spell Guillain-Barré so they could research it."

I was the healthy one, the one my father could count on, but now I've let him down. My mother, my sister, now me. Oh, Dad, what have we done; what have I done to you!

In Cuernavaca, where he lives, the weather is nearly always perfect. Every morning he and my stepmother begin their day in the zocalo with their friends at a table under an umbrella at the Los Arcos Café. They all sip their coffee and watch the action in the square, but my father is the center of attention—always is, always was. Everyone wants him to tell one of his great stories or make some witty remark that will keep them smiling all day. They seldom have long to wait.

There'll be an incident on the street or a person will say something and it will set him going. Mostly his anecdotes are from his life, his childhood in Brooklyn, his years as a newspaperman and as a writer of books and magazine articles. He knew some of the most interesting personalities of his time and his memory is monumental.

"Bob," says Rikki, "I know you're going to be upset, but I've had Marilyn move in with us." Eyes left! Eyes left! Eyes left No! No! No! "Yes," she says, firmly. "I just can't handle everything by myself. I need help."

I feel betrayed, helpless. What can I do? I have lost my

vote. Against my wishes, she's told my parents that I'm sick and she's invited Marilyn. Everyone does to me what they want. "Marilyn will leave just as soon as you come home," she promises. That makes me feel a little better.

Dr. Nagelberg is here. He has a pudgy, pasty face and there is something slimy about him. He's read my x-rays and big surprise—I need another bronchoscopy. He orders Candy to set up the machine. When she asks, with some intensity, which side he'd like it on he's dumbfounded. "What's the difference? Why are you bothering me with that?"

The doctors at Nyack treat the nurses like servants. The nurses seem terrified of them. Aren't they supposed to be professionals? If I used this tone with a professional woman at Texaco, she'd tell me where to stick it.

Dr. Nagelberg is back for the bronchoscopy. "You don't expect me to believe you went skiing in Switzerland by yourself?" he asks Candy.

"Well, I did," she says, handing him a snapshot. He passes it back and she holds it for me to see. I catch a blur of Candy with skis, standing in the snow near a Volkswagen.

"Who took the picture?"

"I did."

"Oh, come on."

"I did. I put the camera on the roof of another car and used the self-timer."

"I don't believe it. You just don't want to tell me who you were shacked up with over there," he says, bumping her hip with his.

No wonder he doesn't care where she has the machine. All he's interested in is getting in her pants. He seems to have about as much chance of that as I do of tap dancing on top of the nurses' station. To put it kindly, he's not Mr. Attractive. He also has zero bedside manner. I only hope his medical skills compensate for his total lack of charm. They've not mentioned anything about morphine. Guess I'm not going to score this time either.

Now he has the instrument and he's holding it up for Candy to see. He wiggles it obscenely. "Think of all the fun a girl could have playing by herself with this," he says. He is a pig.

"Doctor, are you ready?"

"For what?" he leers.

Suddenly, I'm outraged. The son-of-a-bitch wouldn't talk this crudely in front of me if he thought I was more than just a lump of meat; if he knew I could hear, think and remember. Doesn't he know I'll recover? Dr. Fields is often insane but he never forgets I am here. I am me. I AM STILL A PERSON, YOU SLIMY BASTARD!

Anger is a better narcotic than morphine. I fixate on Dr. Nagelberg and not on what he's doing to me. The bronchoscopy seems to be over in a few minutes. Dr. Nagelberg has been grooving on it, but not as intensely as Dr. Fields did.

Candy's bathing me. She's bragging about being invited to lunch at the Peoples' Republic of China's Mission to the United Nations. It is their thanks to her for taking care of a Chinese diplomat who was her patient in the ICU. As she talks, I remember reading that someone deliberately brained the diplomat with a rock as he was enjoying a day at Bear Mountain, a state park. Since it happened soon after the "Red" Chinese opened its mission in New York, it became an embarrassing international incident. Welcome to the U.S.A., honorable diplomat. Conk!

So, Candy was his nurse. I wonder if she flopped down in bed with him, made fun of his body and even the way he talked. The poor bastard probably couldn't even understand what she was saying.

"I visited him in New York at a world famous rehabilitation hospital and do you know what?" she asks me. Eyes left. "He had bed sores. He was here for months and never had a bed sore, but he got one at the world famous hospital.

"Do you like Chinese food?" she wants to know.

Eyes right twice. "Oh, you like it a lot. They say the mission has the best Chinese food in New York. Too bad you're not going to get any," she taunts. Fuck you, bitch!

It's later. It isn't unusual for a patient to change nurses, the head nurse Rikki knows has assured her. "Are you certain you want a different nurse?" Rikki asks me.

The safe thing is to stick with Candy. She's competent and won't accidentally kill me, but she is awful in so many other ways. Having her taken off my case will be a blow to her monumental ego. Yes, I want to do it. She's hurt and humiliated me. I want to get even. Yes, I say again, moving my eyes to the right. "If that's what you want, Darling, I'll tell my friend."

Charlie seems at ease now with the intensive care unit and my situation. The hospital equipment, especially the digital readout of my heart rate, fascinates him. He wants me to see if I can speed it up and slow it down using biofeedback. I try without much success. I don't know if I believe in biofeedback.

Rikki and Charlie have gone and so has Sunday. I'm alone, staring at the ceiling. Without my glasses, I can just make out the pattern of partially plugged holes in the tiles. I try counting them, but I can't concentrate long enough. I hear an alarm off in the distance. I've become so accustomed to the beeps and buzzes that I hardly notice.

Two young men, both doctors, are talking just outside my open curtains. As far as they are concerned, my bed is empty. They don't regard me as a fellow living human being. "You and Gretchen must come sailing with us one weekend this summer," one tells the other.

"You went ahead and bought it, huh?"

"Yeah, we did."

"What did you get, Paul?"

"A 34-foot sloop. It'll sleep four comfortably, six in a pinch."

"I knew you were thinking of a boat but I thought you'd decided to put it off."

"I had, but then I saw an ad for this one, and we looked at it and fell in love, or at least I fell in love. I told Judy the living room furniture could wait a while longer. This is more important."

"I'm jealous. I'm having trouble paying off all my own loans, and you're buying yachts."

"You should have gone into my specialty, my friend. That's where the bucks are," he laughs.

They move on. I don't count. I'm just a thing on a respirator. They don't see the family picture on the wall or the signs Rikki made. They don't know that people love me, that I do count.

I no longer expect to sleep. I've given that up for the duration, along with eating, breathing, sex, fresh air, newspapers, books, music, television and booze. There are times I desperately miss it all, and times I'm lost in thought and forget where I am and what's happened. If they would only turn me more often, my life would be so much easier. Is that so much to ask?

I am thankful Rikki and I had that week in Paris at the end of my trip. It seems strange we ever debated spending the money.

Warren and I were so lucky to have made it to Paris in time for dinner with our wives. All day we knew if things went well with their flights, Rikki and Cathy would be waiting for us at a left bank hotel. We were anxious to tell them all we'd done. We'd been around the world. It had been a great trip, but this had been a hellish day.

Our troubles had started early that morning at the New Delhi airport. The place was a bedlam of pushing, shouting people. You'd think this was their last chance to flee India before the earth swallowed them. The unairconditioned terminal was already hot, dusty and humid. There was no one to tell us what lines we should stand in. What signs there were weren't helpful. They made us fill out complicated forms that made no sense. We were very dumb rats confronting a fiendishly complicated maze.

It had been easy getting into India, but they were making it almost impossible to leave. I've found that many third-world countries joyously welcome you, but they kick and scream when you ask to go home. Because of the airport chaos, our plane was hours late when it finally took off for Rome. Texaco had given us business class tickets for the entire trip, but this huge 747 had no business class. They put us in tourist class and let us know we were lucky to get that.

We were sure we'd missed our connection to Paris, but then we relaxed when we learned that the flight we were on was headed there after a stop in Frankfurt. The only trouble was that it would get us there much too late for dinner with our wives.

Many hours later we were swooping in over Rome. Below was a scene from a travelogue. Golden late afternoon light bathed the city's red tile roofs. I spotted the Coliseum, the Vatican and the Tiber River.

We might not be too late for our connecting flight to Paris after all. It was leaving in ten minutes from the other end of the sprawling terminal. They'd send our luggage to our Paris hotel. There was a chance we could catch the plane. Should we try? "What the hell, let's do it." It was a wild gallop down long corridors. My camera bags bounced on my hips, pulled at my neck, and I had a stitch in my side. "Keep going." I hadn't run this far in years.

Finally, we were at the gates, chests heaving. The plane was ready to go. They'd closed the door, but a charming Italian, an Air France

*employee, made a call. "They're opening the door for us! Italy is a civilized
country! Air France is a wonderful airline!"*

*This flight had no business class so they made us sit in first class.
Pity! We sipped champagne and nibbled French pastries as we watched
the gleaming, snow-covered Alps slip beneath us. This was luxury and
grandeur. I was flying to Paris where the woman I love awaited me. It
was one of the best moments of my life.*

*I adored Paris. Before I ever saw it I worried that I had been
oversold and would be disappointed. But when I finally got there I
realized those fears were groundless. No amount of bad advertising,
schmaltzy songs or terrible movies could ruin this loveliest of cities.*

*Our taxi raced down familiar streets. A couple of years before,
Rikki and I had spent two weeks here. We'd rented bikes for most
of the stay and pedaled all over. It is a great way to learn a city. The
hotel we were heading to was across the Seine from the Louvre. It was
a familiar neighborhood to me, only a half dozen blocks from where
Rikki and I had stayed before. We paid the driver. Were Rikki and
Cathy inside? It would have been such a letdown if not.*

*"They're here!" I saw them sitting in the lobby. Rikki was
reading a guidebook. They jumped up as we came in. We embraced, we
kissed. "How was the trip? You both look so tan, so good," they tell us.
"Where's your luggage?" "In Rome," we laughed, "but don't worry."*

*They had gotten here in the morning, had naps, and been out and
about. "The hotel is fine," they say. Warren and I wanted showers. We
agreed to meet in a half-hour and go out for dinner.*

Kerplunk! Kerplunk! Kerplunk! What the fuck is that
noise? Helen is off tonight. I have some strange nurse who
doesn't even bother to tell me her name. She's so mechanical.
I call her The Robot. I can't even hate her. To get her attention,
I swing my eyes back and forth like a spoiled kid banging his
fist on a table. She reads the list on the poster to find out
what I need. Sometimes I need suctioning, but usually what
I want is turning. "Roll me over in the clover, lay me down

and do it again." She does it a lot. She does it mechanically. What is it she does, you ask? She turns me. I love The Robot.

I'm tired of all this bullshit. I want to get up and go home. Okay, fellas, enough is enough. I've been a good sport up to now, but it's over. I give up. Let me up. I am bored. I am so fucking bored! I'd scream it, if I could.

The terrible sweats have returned. Step right up folks and watch the tube man sweat. He can't talk—he can't even breathe, but boy, can this sucker sweat. Look at the water run off him!

I am sopping wet and so is the bed. The Robot takes note: "He is completely soaked," she says aloud in her mechanical voice. "I must change his linen and bathe him." Good thinking, Robot!

Another bath, another linen change. The Robot's given me one of the best nights I've had, mostly because she doesn't wander off and leave me for long stretches like most other nurses do. And, because she's so mechanical, she's fun to watch. Marry me, Robot. Good night, Robot.

Alice has come on the scene. She tells me that she's my new daytime nurse. Alice is not a Robot. In fact, there is very little distinctive about her aside from her beautiful blue eyes. They don't go with her mousey brown hair. I guess Candy is off the case. Alice doesn't say. It would be unprofessional.

Rikki and Charlie arrive. Today is Monday, they tell me. I know that, for Pete's sake. They check my eyes. No change. They say the phone at home rings constantly with people asking about me and asking if there is anything they can do. "Thank God we have Marilyn to help handle the calls," Rikki says. "People want to visit. Do you want to see anyone?" she asks

No.

"How about Stanley and Dale?"

Yes.

"Do you want your glasses now?" asks Charlie.

No.

"Bob, I had a great idea," he says. "We'll tell everyone who calls that they can leave a message for you on the machine. We'll bring the tape in and play it for you every day. Would you like that?"

Yes, yes!

There are x-rays and blood tests scheduled. Rikki and Charlie must step out. It's the usual agony. There's a fat technician this time. After the x-ray, Dr. Long appears. He's lined up the surgeon for the tracheotomy. "Do you know that Elizabeth Taylor had this operation?" he asks. Will my neck look like hers when it's over?

"It's really a small incision they make in your throat. It's no big deal," he tells me. Why do doctors always say things like this? Wouldn't it be a big deal if it were his throat? "Don't worry about anything," he adds reassuringly. I am not reassured.

~

A physical therapist shows Rikki and Charlie how to put plastic splints on my hands and feet. The ones for the feet are like big ski boots. They're to keep my feet flexed so I don't end up with them pointed down, a condition called foot drop. The hand splints will keep my hands and fingers from curling permanently into a tight ball.

I'm to wear these splints for an hour off and on around the clock. If I don't, the therapist warns, my hands and feet could become frozen in non-functional positions. There is so much that could go wrong with me!

The therapist also shows them how to exercise my arms and legs. Because my IV and other tubes restrict them, they can't move my arms much, but my legs are a different story. He shows them how to bend each one at the knee pushing it back to my chest. And that's pure ecstasy to me. I can't get enough of it.

Dr. Federman interrupts this newfound indulgence. He's come for my daily bronchoscopy. I'd almost forgotten about it. Alice sets up the machine. How will she handle him? Turns out he has no interest in her. "Candy off today?" he asks.

"Yes, she's at some fancy Chinese lunch in New York," she says.

It's late afternoon. Rikki has spoken to Dr. Ramsbotham, the Guillain-Barré specialist in New York. He seems anxious to have me as a patient, she says. He wants to treat me with something called plasmapheresis. It's a way of separating different whole blood components. They have just started using it for Guillain-Barré patients.

He's not terribly optimistic about its doing much good, Rikki says, but he wants to try it. He feels the sooner they do it the better the chances of its working. My case interests him because it is so severe. Plasmapheresis is not dangerous, he says. There is no guarantee it will work, but if it does, it will work quickly.

"Do you want to try it?" Yes, I signal.

"I told him I thought you'd be willing. I'm to call him back later. He may come out to examine you tomorrow." I flash my agreement again. "If he thinks he can help, he'll have you transferred to Columbia-Presbyterian Hospital.

"Okay?" Yes, I answer. Someone might try to treat my problem. Finally, there is some hope, but because the hospital is in Washington Heights, a crime-filled part of the city, I am apprehensive. The neighborhood frightens me and Rikki will be visiting me there. When I lived there as a small child, it was Jewish and solidly lower middleclass. Now it's largely poor and Hispanic.

I'm not indulging in some racist paranoid, suburban fantasy about the big city. I have fresh evidence it's a dangerous neighborhood. Rikki has recently completed a scroll in calligraphy someone ordered as a tribute to a young surgeon murdered on a street near the hospital.

There are always men lurking in doorways in Washington Heights. I won't want Rikki leaving the hospital after dark. But no matter how I fear for Rikki's safety, if they can help me I'll have to go there. The hospital is world-famous. It has some of the nation's best doctors and medical researchers.

I also might have some pull there. One of Texaco's chairman was on the hospital's board and the company has long been a financial supporter.

When Dale had his stroke, he had a large room there with a panoramic view of the Hudson River. It was so different from this tomb. His room was a place to recover; this windowless ward is a place to die.

Charlie has been pumping my legs while Rikki calls Dr. Ramsbotham again. "He's excited by your case," she tells us. "I think I like him, but he sounds strange," she adds without elaboration. I swing my eyes to catch her attention. "Are you asking me why I think he's strange?" Yes. "That's hard to say. He's British, but that's not it. I don't know. I just don't think you'll like him." If he can make me better I don't care if he has two heads.

It's late in the afternoon. We have been waiting hours for the surgeon to do the tracheotomy. "That's the way it is with surgeons," a nurse tells Rikki. "They're always behind schedule."

When we hear that they might put it off until tomorrow, Rikki and Charlie give up and go home. I'm angry. I want it over. Then, suddenly, the two surgeons arrive, instantly turning my anger into fear.

They are slim, good-looking men, very much the modern Europeans. Germans, I guess from their accents. I don't catch their names, so I think of them as Hans and Fritz. They seem oblivious of me, seemingly unaware that I'm awake and watching their every move. They bicker about everything.

"Why did you bring those instruments?" asks Hans. "I wanted the others."

"You didn't say. I am not a mind reader," replies Fritz.

"I don't like operating here."

"Let's get it over and get home. It's late." That's right guys. Slit my throat and hurry on. Dinner's getting cold.

They bark orders at Alice and never say "please." They have her running this way and that. They are going to give me a shot in my neck to deaden the pain. They argue about where it is to go. They compromise and Fritz injects me between the two spots. They wait.

Now Hans has the scalpel. Fritz thinks he should start the incision a little higher. They bicker some more. Has either of them ever done this before? Hans is pushing against my throat with his knife. I feel no pain, just a pressure as if someone is trying to choke me. I hear cartilage ripping. "Shit, look at the blood," says Fritz in amazement. What the fuck was he expecting?

They're trying to stop the bleeding and they're yelling at Alice to get them things. Through the din I hear the PA system calling for the owners of a Porsche and a Mercedes, both with MD license plates, to immediately move their cars or have them towed away. I instantly know that the cars belong to Hans and Fritz.

"Call the operator!" Hans orders Alice, "Tell her we're in the middle of an emergency operation. We'll move the cars when we're done."

"Why is he bleeding so much?" Fritz asks her when she returns.

"Maybe because he's on Heparin," Alice meekly guesses.

"Heparin!" roars Hans. "Why didn't someone tell us?"

They've stopped the bleeding, but not their squabbling. Where is that famed German cool? Now they're yanking the breathing tube I've had in my throat. I'm expecting the terrible sore throat Stanley described, but if I have one I can't feel it. Maybe it's because I can't swallow.

They are gathering their things to leave. Everything is okay. "We'll be back tomorrow to remove the packing," they promise.

They're gone. I see four tiny brown spots on the ceiling tile that I hadn't noticed before. Are they new? Did my blood squirt up there and cause them? I cannot tell.

It's night and The Robot is back on duty. Good thing too. I'm again a fountain of mucus. Need suctioning all the damn time. The Robot attends me well, but tonight she ignores my pleas to be turned. It's as though she can only handle one problem at a time.

I'm fantasizing about Columbia-Presbyterian, imagining rows of beautiful rooms, each looking out at the Hudson and the George Washington Bridge. This is New York, the big leagues. All the nurses are friendly and coolly professional. All the doctors are sane. Best part of all, every twenty minutes teams of attendants go from room to room, turning patients.

Kerplunk! Kerplunk! No sleep. I stare at the spots on the ceiling. My blood? There's no way to know. For years to come, other patients will wonder about those spots.

I'm dying of discomfort again. I flash my eyes at The Robot. The Robot does not read my signal. Move me, move me instantly, you dumb fucking Robot!

Jesus, now what? Something new and frightening—a loud gurgling fills my head. I can't get anyone's attention, but if I do, how do I tell them what's wrong? My problem is not on Rikki's list. Is there something wrong with the respirator? Is the dumb thing going to crap out? Is it a Ralph Nader special?

Now every time the machine pumps another breath, there's this roaring in my head. It's as loud as an express racing through a local subway station. The sound terrifies me. It could be killing me. Help me, please! Someone tell me what's going on.

Kerplunk! Well, I'm not dead yet. The Robot has come and suctioned and turned me and read the list to me. I keep shifting my eyes to say no and she can't figure out what's wrong. Poor, confused Robot. Will I live with this fucking noise forever? I'll go deaf and maybe blind, as Rikki fears. I'll end up worse off than Helen Keller. She at least could walk and use her arms.

A respiratory technician is here to change some part of the machine. I flash him my signal, eyes back and forth. He listens for a moment, and then does something under my neck, shutting off the sound completely. "I'm sorry Bob," he says. "That shouldn't have happened." What shouldn't have happened? I can't ask.

Another night is ending. Maybe one of the last I'll have to endure here. The Robot is leaving. "Goodbye," she says in her mechanical voice. "I am off tonight. You'll have someone else."

Now I have another thing to worry about. Who will they give me tonight? The Robot and I were working things out. I'll have some new nurse who doesn't know me, who will have to learn so much. There is no peace.

Rikki and Charlie are here. It cheers me just to see them. "We brought the tape, Bob," says, Charlie. "Should I play it?" Yes. The first call is from Wanda, saying they miss me. Then the voices of friend after friend, all saying it differently, but all telling me they care. There are calls from people I work with and old friends—it's wonderful to hear them.

I signal Charlie. I want him to exercise my legs, but he doesn't understand. He stops the tape and runs through the list, trying to find what I want. The exercises aren't on the poster. He goes through the list again, thinking he may have missed something. Then he remembers the exercises.

"Is that what you want?" Yes. "Did I hit the jackpot, Bob?" Yes.

Charlie pumps my legs as I listen to the last of the calls, including one from Warren who makes a joke about me noticing a pretty nurse. Charlie must have told him that I looked at her when he was here. "I'm glad that part of you wasn't affected," he says with a chuckle.

My father's familiar gravelly voice is next. His Brooklyn accent is more noticeable on tape. He's uncomfortable speaking to a machine. Since it's Rikki's recorded voice that has answered, he talks to her. If she needs them, he says, they'll fly up immediately. They're sending us $1,000. They'll try to send more if we're short of money. The machine partially cuts his message off before he finishes. Nothing as insignificant as a beep-tone could ever shut him up.

"I called them back right away," says Rikki, "and told them there was no need for them to come. That you had specifically asked that they not come."

Yes!

"I also told them not to send any more money."

Yes!

I'm crying again. We don't need their money. $1,000 is a significant sum to them. They have no savings, only a small income from Social Security, and the interest from a certificate of deposit, which they bought (at my urging) with money my sister left them in her life insurance. Louise also receives a pension from Time-Life, where she worked for many years as a researcher.

As a freelance writer, my father had good years and lean years. During the poor years he felt deprived, so when a good one came along he was like a sailor hitting port after months at sea. Better blow it all now. Never know when you'll see land again. He and Louise never saved a dime—thought it small and cheap to save money, something ribbon clerks did.

One year he sent Charlie $10 for Christmas. He could barely wait to ask me what Charlie had done with the dough. "He put it in the bank," I told him.

"In the bank?" he asked, incredulous. "Why would he do that?" He was mystified. If Charlie had blown it all on nonsense, he would have understood. In fact, he would have been delighted. But why would a kid want to save money in a bank?

Sometimes, just to tease, I demand my inheritance. "It's so unfair to make me sit around and wait all these years," I wail. "Why can't I have at least some of it now?" He shakes with laughter. He knows I know there will be no inheritance. I don't love him for his money.

I want instant recovery. I want to talk to my father. I want to return all the phone calls, thank everyone for their concern, tell them it's okay, I'm all better now. I'll be back at work in a couple of days. I'm available for Christmas parties.

Dr. Long has joined us. He has spoken with Dr. Ramsbotham and Dr. Ramsbotham wants me as a patient.

"Do you think we should make the move?" asks Rikki, suddenly tearful. "I don't know what to do. Tell me what we should do." The pressure is getting to her now.

"There are no hard answers," he says, "but yes, I think you should go. Plasmapheresis could work. It's certainly worth trying. However, there is risk in a move like this for someone in Bob's condition."

"Would you take it?" Rikki wants to know.

"I think I would, but how do you feel about it, Bob? Do you want to make the move?" Yes, I signal. Yes. I want to get out of here. I want to get better as fast as possible.

Charlie looks tired. He's exercising my legs, pumping them back and forth. I can't get enough. It's hard work for him. My legs are muscular and heavy. He keeps at it, finally asking if it's enough. Yes, I signal, but in truth there's no such thing as enough when it comes to moving my legs.

Rikki is putting on my hand splints. I can't move a muscle, but the splints make me feel powerful. They remind me of the equipment offensive football linemen wear. Next, she fastens the splints to my feet. The plastic digs painfully into them.

"Rikki! They told us never to do it tight!" Charlie shouts, ripping away the Velcro straps.

"Whatever I do is wrong. I can't do anything right," she sobs. Rikki is so hard on herself. She drives herself constantly to succeed, to avoid feeling like a failure. It sometimes makes her difficult to live with.

She's alone in her low self-appraisal. Everyone else sees her as managing things so well. She thinks they don't know the real her, but I know the real her. This morning has been a good example of what she does without giving herself credit. Without any fuss, she's made all the arrangements for the move into the city. Everything is set. Rikki pushes herself.

Dr. Federman has completed another bronchoscopy and seems elated. Nothing modest about his ego. I wonder how much the bastards make from each one of these. No, I know better. I'm not that cynical. They do them because it's needed, not to make money.

Dale and Stanley share a strong faith in the expertise that's available in the city. They're relieved that I'm moving to a New York hospital. Stanley is taking the morning off from his practice to drive Rikki down. There won't be enough room for her in the ambulance.

It's late in the afternoon and Rikki and Charlie talk about going home. Before they can, Dr. Schwartz, my neurologist, joins us. He's sorry I'm leaving Nyack but he knows we want a larger hospital. I note his impeccable black suit.

"Move your leg," he orders. I try but there's not even a tremor.

"You have to make yourself move! You have to try!" he says with the fervency of a backwoods preacher. "Now move your leg. Tell yourself you're going to move it."

"You can do it, Bob, you can do it!" Charlie chimes in.

"That's right son, he has to try. He has to have the desire."

Have the desire! How does this bastard dare suggest I lack desire? If that's all it took, I would have fled this fucking mad house long ago. Don't you remember? You told me I have an electrical problem; the circuits are out. The insulation is burnt off the wires. The call won't go through. "Sorry, your call cannot be completed. Please hang up." My brain has been disconnected.

"You can do it, Bob!" Charlie choruses, as if cheers will make me rise. If I could do it, I'd tell Dr. Schwartz where to stick it. How can a man who made such a brilliant diagnosis imply that all that's wrong now is my lack of desire? He's laying the blame on me. He's saying it's my fault, not his. It's nobody's fault, you asshole!

Good news! Jenny is my nurse. A gift from the Gods. My last night here and I have someone who is good and who realizes I'm a human. What relief.

"You have a visitor," Jenny says. I signal no, I don't want a visitor. Stanley and Dale and Rikki and Charlie have been here. There's no one else I want to see.

But Jenny misses my protest. Dean Francis and his son, Alexander, a boy in his last year of high school, appear. Alex is intimidated by what he sees and hangs back, but Dean comes close.

I had forgotten about Dean. He could have been on the list of those I'd let visit. His Minnesota boyhood was shaped by a series of terrible operations to correct a birth defect in his stomach. He's been an intensive care patient many times. He knows the nakedness I feel being here.

"I had to come when I heard," he says, in a voice so quiet I can barely make out what he's saying. "This is the first chance I had." I shift my eyes to the right to show I understand, but he doesn't know about my signals.

"It's awful when they have you hooked up to all the tubes. I hate those. The nose tube's the worst. I couldn't stand that." I stare up at him with my blurred vision. He's so hard to see and hear. "Well, we should go. Good luck," he says, softly touching my hand.

I feel a few tears. I'd love to tell him, "Pick me up at 7:30, okay?" For years I commuted to the city with Dean in his various rusting Volkswagens. That stopped when Texaco moved out to the suburbs. Now we don't see each other often.

As they bathe me, Jenny and another young nurse, keep up a lively chatter. I'm included in the conversation. They talk about the coming holidays. Will I be home for Christmas, I wonder.

"Was that your son I saw?" Jenny asks. Yes. "He's cute." She guesses his age and is disappointed to learn he's only nineteen. "Too young for me."

"But Jenny you're engaged," says the other girl.

"That's why I have to fool around now," she snaps back. "Pretty soon I won't be able to."

When they're done with my bath she tells me, "You still look like you've been on a three-day drunk, Mr. Samuels. Have you been shaved since you've been here?" No.

"Well, I'm going to shave you. Can't have you going to the big city in that condition."

I'm freshly bathed and shaved and comfortably lying on my side. For the moment, I'm a contented man. I'm anxious for the new day and the new hospital. Too bad I didn't have a marvelous nurse like Jenny the whole time I was here. It would have made a huge difference.

Life's so often like that: a big crapshoot. Random luck brings an individual sperm to an egg, not to mention the chance that brings a father to a mother.

We make many choices, but the important stuff seems to happen on its own. It's as though we're all on small individual rafts, bobbing down a wide river. The water is calm and blue. We steer this way and that, sometimes even briefly paddling against the flow, seemingly in control. But the current pushes us relentlessly on. Unexpectedly, the river can narrow and suddenly the rapids are upon us. It's all white water now and we have no control. Tremendous boulders threaten. If our luck holds, if random chance is with us and our raft isn't smashed on a rock or sucked into a whirlpool, we reach the next run of blue water.

The river sets everyone a different course. Some seem to miss the rapids completely—others never see calm. But the river flows in the same direction for us all. Eventually, it's over the falls and into the abyss for everyone.

The mucus, the damn mucus has flooded me again and Jenny is here suctioning. She is barely away from my bed when the terrible sweats hit once more. I need another bath. I'm like an infant. I need constant care.

The young respiratory care technician is explaining that the ambulance doesn't have a respirator. I'll have to be ambued by hand all the way down. He detaches the respirator hose from the trach tube in my neck to show me what that means. In its place puts the plastic end of the ambu. It looks like a small, soft, roundish football.

He squeezes the ambu and a breath of air fills my lungs. With each squeeze, there's another breath. "I think they're going to assign me to go with you," he says, trying to conceal his excitement. To him there's drama in the ambulance ride and the trip to the big city hospital.

Things are happening quickly now. Rikki and Charlie have arrived with Stanley. They all keep looking at their watches. A pale, heavy-set nurse with bleached hair is going to ride with me. I don't like her. The young respiratory technician isn't coming with us after all. Instead, they've given the job to another technician, a short, stocky, no-nonsense young woman. I immediately trust her. She'll have my life in her hands—literally.

Dr. Long is here to say goodbye. "Let us know how you're doing," he says, "and come by and see us when you're home."

Dr. Federman is here now too. He's ticked off. No one has told him I was leaving. "I hope they know down there that he needs a bronchoscopy every day or he won't make it," he says.

The ambulance has arrived. Everyone is shooed away while I'm slid onto a narrow stretcher, covered with heavy blankets and strapped down. I'm rolling through a corridor, the ambu girl in step beside me. There's Charlie, Rikki and Stan. As I reach the door, I see Rikki fling herself sobbing into Stanley's arms.

The outside air is a shock. It's turned so cold. The head of the stretcher jerks. I'm in the ambulance. The doors slam shut.

I'm surprised how cramped it is. The ambu girl and the nurse sit squeezed together on a bench facing me. There wouldn't have been room for Rikki. Hope she's okay. No siren—this isn't considered an emergency, I suppose.

We're rolling south on 9W, retracing the route Rikki and I took last week. Has it just been a week? It seems so much longer. I wish I could look out and not just up. All I see are the bare tops of trees, stark against a slate winter sky, but I know just where we are. There's a sweeping view of the Hudson from here this time of year.

Soon we'll pass the turnoff for our street. I'm homesick for everything there. It's as though I've been gone months. All I want now is home. I long for it, ache for it. I know that house better than I know my own body. It is old, begun before the Revolutionary War and in the fourteen years we've lived there, every part of it has needed my attention.

Maybe Rikki has asked them to stop at the house. If they open the back doors of the ambulance, I'd be able to see it. They could let Ruffy into the ambulance. I'll cry if I see him. He'll lick my face. Poor old Ruff dog, going blind, getting old. Tears are filling my eyes. Jesus, think of something else. Don't cry now.

We're stopping for a red light at the turnoff for our road. They'd say something to each other if we were going to the house. We're not turning. I must remember that my life's at stake. They can't fool around. A girl is squeezing a bag to keep me breathing.

I trust her. She doesn't miss a beat. What if something goes wrong? We could stop at hospitals along the way, but I think we only pass one in Englewood, New Jersey.

Now we're climbing the hill in Palisades. We're passing our swim club where Rikki and I have lazed away many hot summer days. This hill is a bitch, steep and endless. I've struggled up it with my bike the few times I've peddled to the city. On the rock cut near the top you can still see the message, "The Kid loves Pook," that someone painted years ago.

One late night, tired and drunk, I told my friends, "You realize, of course, 'The Kid loves Pook.'" I didn't expect anyone to know what in hell I was talking about, but everyone did and everyone thought they alone had noticed the graffiti.

"The question is," said one of my friends, "who is The Kid?"

"No, no," said someone else. "The real question is who is Pook?"

"Not who is, what is?"

"And why does the kid love her/it?"

"Maybe we all love her or it?"

Even though I can't see the message, I know it is there, an enigma for commuters to ponder each morning.

Does The Kid remember painting the rocks? Does he ever drive by to see how it's weathered? Did he marry Pook and have children, or did she break his heart? Does she see the sign and wish she'd stuck with The Kid? How does this novel end?

Time to get me off this side! Time to move! The bumps of the road are killing me. It feels as though there's a terrible weight pressing me, gravity gone berserk. I can't tolerate the pain. I have to move! I'm shifting my eyes back and forth to get their attention. The ambu girl notices immediately and alerts the nurse.

"What's wrong, honey?" she asks. "You uncomfortable?"

Yes, yes, thank God you know what I want. You're not so bad. I was wrong about you. I adore you. You're lovely.

"I can't do anything for you until we get to the hospital. I can't move you"

Yes you can, you dumb fucking cow! You think you're just along for the ride? You're supposed to take care of me. Move me now, bitch! I shift my eyes furiously.

"You're strapped down. I can't move you. You'll have to wait until we're at the hospital."

"We're almost to the Parkway," says the ambu girl.

Don't tell me where we are. I know exactly where we are and it's not even halfway to the hospital. I can't make it the rest of the way.

We're slowing for the left turn and now we're on the Parkway. Christ, we'll never get there. I'm so weak. I can't stand it. Jesus, it's so painful. Oh God, fuck this. MOVE ME NOW! I scream with my eyes.

"Mr. Samuels, I can't move you," the nurse, The Cow, says, firmly. "You're strapped down."

Loosen the straps! What's so holy about the fucking straps? You think I don't feel pain because I'm paralyzed. I feel just like you do. I'm shifting my eyes as fast as I can.

"I'm not going to move you. I can't," insists the nurse.

I won't make it. I will die before we get there. The pain is unbearable. The stretcher is as hard as a marble slab; the pillows propping me are granite. Every bounce, every jolt slams through me.

At this hour it's usually a fifteen-minute shot down the Parkway to the George Washington Bridge. Today it seems endless. I've driven this Parkway since it opened in the 1950s. I've been on it night and day, in every kind of weather. It tops the New Jersey palisades cliffs, high above the Hudson River. It is a safe road, a beautiful road, but there have been times up here when I sensed death was waiting for me.

I was stranded alone one night in a heavy snow on the Parkway and thought death was there to meet me. But soon I realized that I was wrong, that I wasn't going to freeze, that night. The inside of my VW was cold but not that cold. I relaxed. I even became bored. At daylight three beefy guys in a Buick came along and gave me a lift to a shopping center.

But death lurks here on nights when milk dense fogs rise from the river. You follow the white curb blindly and hope no fool without lights is stopped ahead. The white curb is all you have.

That curb has saved my life. As a young reporter working the lobster shift at Brooklyn police headquarters, I often drove home exhausted. Sometimes I'd doze and the car would drift to the right. It would hit the corrugated surface of that curb, jolting me awake in terror.

Now I know death is here. No curb will save me; no rescuers will come. I'm tired, so tired. I'm meeting death and I'm glad. There will be no more pain.

I'm drenched. The terrible sweats have begun. If only the sweat could grease me enough so I'd slide on this marble slab. The nurse and the ambu girl look worried about me. That's good. If I keep sweating and flashing, maybe they'll realize they have to help me. Take me to Englewood Hospital. Get me off this fucking stretcher. Let me move. Lift the terrible weight. Oh, please!

"We're close to the Englewood exit," says the driver. My spirits soar. They must be planning to stop at the hospital. Roll me around on a hospital bed. Just ten minutes, five minutes. That's all I ask. Even one minute. Anything!

Am I out of my mind? They're not going to stop just to move me around—or are they? Why would the driver even mention the Englewood exit if we weren't getting off? He's not conducting a tour.

Maybe the nurse gave him a signal. The patient is in trouble! Get to Englewood Hospital quick. No siren, though. Cool it and don't scare him.

Fuck it, man. Use the siren. Pour it on. Let it sing. Won't scare me.

He's not turning. We're going straight ahead and I'm going to die. I can't move, can't talk, can't breath. I ought to die. I deserve to die. That's why Nyack was so willing to let me go. Let the sucker die in somebody else's hospital.

"I'll do that for a while," says the nurse. "You need a break." She wants the ambu. Don't let her have it. Don't give her the football! She won't squeeze it the right way, not like you. You're so even and steady. I know you're tired, but please don't give her the football.

"That's all right," says the ambu girl. "It's my job."

"You're tired. I won't mind doing it."

"No, I'll do it. Thanks."

We're slowing. Must be for the bridge. "Anyone have money for the toll?" asks the driver. He has to be kidding. I know it's a joke. We're through the toll so he was kidding.

Now we're into the long curve of the ramp. It's bumpy and hard, awful. Loosen the straps. Get me off this side. Please, I beg of you. Please, you bastards, please.

I love all bridges, but especially this one. When I was a small boy in Washington Heights, it was part of the landscape, as familiar as the local playground. That was forty years ago and the bridge looked shiny new then. The name, The George Washington Bridge, sounded so dignified and important, so fitting. Now the bridge is old and grey, more dignified and more important than ever and even more deserving of its name.

If I get to the hospital, I want a room overlooking the bridge and the river. The Hudson marks one of the divisions within me. I've been half city boy and half suburban most of my life. The river symbolizes the split and the bridge connects the parts.

I will die in the center of the bridge and no one will understand the symbolism. Fuck symbolism! I don't want to die. Jesus, just get me across the bridge and onto a bed. We're so close. The pain will stop once I move. Rikki will be there. She'll help me. Charlie will pump my legs. Jesus, imagine having my legs moved!

But I won't make it. I'll never see them again. We're going to get lost. Columbia-Presbyterian is in many buildings. No chance this joker will locate the right one. We're less than five minutes away, but it could take him a half hour to find it. I'll die on some crummy Washington Heights street.

"We're on Broadway. It won't be long now," says the driver.

"Do you know which building it is?" asks the ambu girl.

"Yeah, I asked before we left. It's easy to get lost down here."

"We'll be there in a couple of minutes," the nurse says, stroking my forehead. I have my doubts.

We're stopping. The attendant runs out to check if this is the building. He's back in a moment. "This is it. We're here," he reports.

~

It happens fast. I'm out of the ambulance, through some swinging doors and into the hospital. Now we're on an elevator, now in a corridor. I miss details. The ambu girl is with me. Couldn't breathe otherwise. Now they're sliding me onto a bed. Oh Jesus, it feels so good.

An excitable little guy named Vinnie is helping. He has me hooked to a respirator. Suddenly they're all gone. It's just him and me. He's upset, cursing in Italian. Pale light comes through the filthy window. The room is cramped. One side of the bed is against the wall, with a sink at the foot. The walls are an institutional green and peeling. It all reminds me of a terrible little room we stayed in one night in Bologna, Italy.

The respirator at Nyack was at the head of the bed, out of my line of sight. Here it's alongside the bed. Each time it pumps a breath, I see the bellows move. The machine, like everything else here, is beat-up and grimy.

Vinnie curses the people who brought me here. He asks, with his eyes cast toward heaven, why they didn't suction me. He yanks a suctioning tube from its sealed glassine paper wrappings. It's the same noisy paper they use on the slim bags for Italian bread sticks.

When he's done, there's little to throw away. Every time they suctioned me in Nyack it left a big pile of plastic junk, like the remains of a meal at McDonald's.

Vinnie is an artist with the suction catheter. He has a talent for it. In every way he's a superb nurse, the best I've had. He's fast, even frantic, but he's always gentle with the patient. I know I'm completely safe with him. Moving to New York was the right decision.

I hear Rikki and Charlie in the hall. Vinnie orders them in. Everything agitates him. I like him a lot.

"Lady," Vinnie tells Rikki, "you got to go to the registry and tell them you need private duty nurses."

"Okay," Rikki says, but I can tell she hasn't really heard him. She's looking for a place on the wall to put the checklist and the sign about me answering with my eyes. She doesn't like the room. Who would? It's as ugly as can be.

"You want me to exercise your legs?" asks Charlie. Yes. Yes. That's just what I want. "Did I hit the jackpot?" Yes, yes!

"Did you like the ambulance ride?" No.

Stanley is here. "Everything all right?" he asks.

Everything's fine, Rikki tells him. "They didn't exactly give you the luxury suite, did they?" Stan jokes. The room is so small that he, Rikki and Charlie fill it.

"Now that I know you're safe," he says, "I'm going to work." Rikki walks him to the elevator. It was so generous of him to take off from his practice.

"What was wrong with the ambulance?" Charlie asks when we're alone. He's still pumping my legs. I swing my eyes to remind him that I can't answer essay questions, only true/false.

"Was it really terrible?"

Yes.

"Was it the worst ride you every had to New York?"

Yes.

"Did you think you might die?"

Yes.

"Bob thought he might die in the ambulance," Charlie tells Rikki as she comes back to the room.

"Oh, darling, did you?"

Yes, I sure did.

There's someone here. God, she's a beautiful young Italian-American woman—tall, dark and slim. Her name is Dr. Rossi and she's the resident for this floor. Rikki and Charlie must wait outside while she examines me.

If they told me they'd transferred me to a hospital in Rome, I might believe it. I could be in a time warp. It's as unsettling as an episode of "The Twilight Zone." Everything's Italian—the staff, room, the paper on the catheter—all very convincing.

I hope that the room is temporary. It's unimportant now but I don't want anyone visiting me here. I'm pathetic enough as it is.

Dr. Rossi is very bright. She has immediately caught on to my eye signals. Vinnie is helping her turn me for the examination. To get around the bed, they must shove it away from the wall. The examination is thorough. No part of me is private any longer. When they're finished, I hear Vinnie in the hall again reminding Rikki to hire nurses.

"Will you tell me all about the ambulance ride when you're able to talk?" Charlie asks.

Yes, I promise, yes.

"Are you glad we came here?" Rikki asks. Yes.

"If you don't like it here we can have you moved to another hospital," she says.

No! This building would have to be on fire before I'd leave. The trip from Nyack almost killed me! Don't you understand?

"Yes, we can," she insists, her voice edging out of control. "We can go to any hospital in the city—any hospital in the world that will make you better soon."

No! No! No!

"But we can. You understand that? We can!"

Yes, I understand. But I can't survive them moving me again. Let's see what these people can do. Give them a chance.

"Mrs. Samuels?" asks an English accented voice.

"Yes."

"I'm Dr. Ramsbotham." I stare up at him in amused amazement. He's a British eccentric right out of a loopy comedy. His graying hair shoots from his skull like a man with a finger stuck in a light socket. He has kind blue eyes and rough pale skin. His nose is a raw red, making him look like he has a permanent cold. He's tall so his ample pot and wide hips aren't immediately apparent. A loud, cheap tie is around his neck. I'd guess he's in his late fifties.

"How are you feeling, sir?" he asks politely. I flash him a yes.

"Does your husband communicate at all?" he asks Rikki.

"Yes," she says, explaining how I move my eyes for yeses and nos. Charlie grabs the sign from the wall to show him.

"All right, I'll try again. How are you feeling, sir?" he repeats, as if I hadn't understood the question the first time. Yes, I answer.

"What does that mean?" he wants to know.

"Bob's saying yes," Rikki explains. "I guess it means he's feeling okay. Try to ask questions that have yes or no answers. Let me show you. Are you feeling all right?" she asks. I instantly flash another yes.

"See how well that works?" Charlie says enthusiastically.

"Yes, yes?" he replies uncertainly. "I'd like to examine you, sir." he says. Yes, I flash. "Did that mean yes?" he asks Rikki.

"That's right," she says, brightening. "You're catching on."

Dr. Ramsbotham is examining me by himself. He's very timid and polite, far too gentle to turn me on my side, as he should. The beautiful Dr. Rossi joins us. She's trying to save him time by giving him her findings but he's not listening. He thinks she's a nurse. At first she doesn't grasp his misunderstanding. When she finally catches on, she's furious.

She's drifted away but he's hardly noticed. Vinnie now is here helping, rolling me on my side. Dr. Ramsbotham seems to be puttering around. His upper-class English disdain for Vinnie is obvious to me, but Vinnie seems not to notice.

"What happened to the nurse?" Dr. Ramsbotham asks him.

"What nurse? I'm the nurse."

"You're the nurse?" He's incredulous. He thinks Vinnie must be an attendant. "That young lady who was here—where did she go?"

"Young lady? Oh, you mean Dr. Rossi. I don't know where she went."

The examination is over. Dr. Ramsbotham has summoned Rikki and Charlie back into the room. He tells them he's asking Dr. Schick, a colleague who specializes in lung problems, and Dr. Fittipaldi, the man who's in charge of plasmapheresis, and a urologist whose name I don't catch, all to look at me.

"Is this the best that can be done for Bob?" asks Charlie.

"We're certainly going to try our best."

"What are the chances that the plasmapheresis will work?"

"It's experimental."

"Just what does that mean?" says Charlie, going after him like Mike Wallace chasing a sleazy Florida real estate developer around a parking lot. I've never seen Charlie so aggressive.

"It means we don't know how well it will work." I expect Dr. Ramsbotham to lose his temper at any moment.

"Can it do any harm?"

"We don't believe so."

"Don't you know?"

"Not positively."

"Could Bob die?"

"Not from the plasmapheresis."

"When will you start the treatments?"

"Very soon."

"Not today?"

"No."

"I want the best treatment for my father. Do you understand? I want the very best."

"Of course."

Charlie's assertiveness both embarrasses and surprises me. We're here because Dr. Ramsbotham is New York's top Guillain-Barré specialist. Charlie knows that. He should give him some respect.

The day is passing. I hear Vinnie bitching in the hall to someone about Rikki not hiring nurses. Finally, he bursts in. "Lady, if you don't go across to the registry right now and tell them your husband needs a nurse for the night, you're not going to get one." Finally, Rikki hears him. She's leaving for the registry.

I wonder why the regular hospital nurses can't take care of me.

Oh, Jesus, they're here for x-rays. I dread this. Vinnie is helping the technician, a woman. No problem. They roll me on my side toward the wall, then back on the plate. Why couldn't they have been this gentle at Nyack?

Rikki is back. She got to the registry just before it closed. They are sending a nurse for tonight and looking for one for tomorrow. I'll need two nurses working twelve-hour shifts, or three on eight-hour shifts. Either way the cost is three hundred dollars a day and you have to pay it daily.

"Don't worry, darling," she says. "The registry woman said insurance usually covers most of it." I want to ask why we must hire our own nurses.

Charlie is leaving. He's taking my car back to school. I don't like that but no one bothers to ask my opinion. What if the plasmapheresis works and I'm completely better by next week? Then I'll need the car to get to work and he'll have to drive it all the way back from Maryland.

Rikki has left us alone to say our goodbyes. "You're going to get better soon," Charlie says, holding my hand.

Yes!

"The plasmapheresis will work."

Yes!

"You'll make a complete recovery."

Yes!

He bends to kiss me. "I love you Bob," he whispers. I love you my son. Fresh tears fill my eyes.

He's out the door and gone. Then, suddenly, I hear him again. "You can do it, Bob, you can do it," he calls through the door.

Pearl is my evening nurse. She's very passive, one of those sexless women between 35 and 55 who drift through life without men, without any real friends. Everything about her is vague and tentative. Even her race is uncertain. She appears to be mostly Caucasian, but then, in certain lights, she seems black or even Asian.

Rikki is telling her everything about me at once. It would be difficult for anyone to follow her. Pearl maintains a thin, pleasant smile. She nods while Rikki talks, as if she understands everything. I have my doubts, but it doesn't matter. Pearl's a registered nurse. She'll know what to do. She doesn't need Rikki's instructions. This is Columbia-Presbyterian Hospital—one of the best. They wouldn't send anyone untrained.

"Do you have children?" Rikki asks, trying as always to establish a human bond.

"I have a son."

"That's nice. Does he live with you?"

"No, he's married. He lives in Rochester."

"So you and your husband are alone?"

"I don't have a husband." She offers no details.

Rikki is getting ready to go home. Do I want her to come back later tonight? No. If you don't count the time it takes to park, the hospital is less than a half-hour from our house.

"Then I'll see you early in the morning, my darling." Yes. "You'll be okay with Pearl?" Yes.

It's been at least a half-hour since Rikki left. I need to be suctioned. It's not an emergency, not urgent but I want to test Pearl, know how she works. So far she's done nothing for me, just talked with Rikki. I swing my eyes back and forth, but I'm facing the wall. I don't see Pearl. Maybe she's not here, not in the room. I haven't heard her since Rikki left. I listen carefully. All I hear is the respirator. I feel deserted, desolate. · Why did I let Rikki leave me with this strange creature in this horrible room?

This is the first time since I arrived that I haven't been able to tell Charlie or Rikki to get Vinnie to suction me. It won't occur to Vinnie to check on me now. He knows I have a nurse.

What would happen if it were an emergency, if I needed help? Wait! There's a shadow. "Mr. Samuels?" A beautiful Asian face peers down at me. "Mr. Samuels, I'm Dr. Schick. Dr. Ramsbotham asked me to come by and take care of your lungs."

A young colleague is with her. "Don't worry, sir," he says dramatically. "We will make you better." What a jackass he is. Now I see Pearl. She's standing behind them.

They're going to do a bronchoscopy. The x-rays show I'm drowning again. They roll in a machine that looks even older than the one in Nyack. I'm not surprised. Everything here is beat-up.

Dr. Schick wants Pearl to suction me. Pearl is slow, awkward with the suction. Jesus, she's awful. She's jamming the tube in my mouth, then up my nose.

"Always suction the nose first, then the mouth," Dr. Schick tells her. "It's more sterile that way. If you suction the mouth first, you should change catheters before doing the nose."

I wasn't aware of that, but as she says it I realize that's the way every nurse has done it. Shouldn't Pearl have known that? My faith in her is wobbling.

"We'll need a consent for the bronchoscopy," Dr. Rabins, Dr. Schick's young colleague, reminds her. Rikki can't sign. She's gone home, Pearl tells them.

"Can Mr. Samuels communicate at all?" Dr. Schick asks.

"I don't think so," replies Pearl.

You don't think so, you dumb bitch. Rikki explained repeatedly how I answer questions.

"Look here," Dr. Schick's assistant says, pointing at the poster, "it says he can answer yes and no by moving his eyes.

"Mr. Samuels, you know what a bronchoscopy is?" I flash him an instant yes. "Do we have your permission to go ahead with the procedure?" Yes, again. Go to it. Don't hesitate. At Nyack, Dr. Federman said if I didn't have one every day I'd die.

Damn! No morphine. Not even a mention. If they don't give it to me for the first bronchoscopy, they never will.

I don't know why doctors find bronchoscopies so exciting but Dr. Schick is into it. She's giving us a running narrative of her travels through my lungs: "Upper right lobe, lower left lobe...."

We have good friends named Loeb. I start naming my Loebs as she names hers. There's Werner Loeb, his wife, Nedra Loeb, and their children, Susan Loeb, Janice Loeb, and Chuck Loeb. Susan and Janice have both been married. Are they still Loebs? I must ask Werner. It's a legal question and he's a lawyer. He ought to know.

"Look at this junk, just look at it," Dr. Schick says angrily. Why is she so mad? Is it someone's fault?

She offers Dr. Rabins and Pearl a chance to view my lungs through the instrument. He grabs for it but she declines. She's indifferent to everything.

I'm erupting with mucus. Suction, suction! Pearl can't get it together. It's all overwhelming her! First, she has to don a sterile glove, attach a suctioning catheter to a tube and open a valve. Only at that point should she disconnect the respirator hose to my neck. She then must move quickly to suction me. Until she reattaches the hose, I'm without air.

If she goes too slowly, the respirator begins beeping annoyingly. The noise upsets her, makes her fumble. She can turn it off by flipping a day-glow orange switch.

"But if you turn it off," Dr. Schick cautions, "you must remember to turn it on again or it could be very dangerous. If the switch is up, the alarm won't beep even if the hose is accidentally disconnected." Shouldn't Pearl already know this?

I should have chest p.t. every couple of hours, Dr. Schick tells Pearl. In the Air Force, p.t. meant physical training, calisthenics. I can't imagine what Dr. Schick is talking about. She demonstrates. She yanks the sheet off, pulls my hospital gown up, and starts rhythmically beating on my ribs with her cupped hands. I'm astonished. I feel like a drum. "This will loosen the congestion in his lungs," she says.

It's Pearl's turn. She has very small hands. She pounds one side of my chest, then turns me the other way and pounds the other side. It doesn't hurt. In fact, I rather enjoy it. Anything to have my body moved.

Dr. Schick and Dr. Rabins have been gone for quite a while. Dr. Schick seems nice. Chinese maybe, in her forties. Not a very Chinese name but I gather it's a married name.

I've had my eye drops. Hope they help. My vision is lousy. Don't think I can sleep. Haven't slept for over a week. So strange. What time is it now?

I need suctioning again. Pearl sits on the room's one chair gazing into space. Somehow I catch her eye and she gets my message and rises. She detaches the hose from my neck. The respirator starts beeping like a bulldozer in reverse. The noise flusters her. Doesn't she realize that I can't breathe without the respirator? My hands tingle from lack of oxygen. My vision dims. Hurry! Please hurry!

"Is everything okay in here?" a young man asks. He sees what's wrong, pushes Pearl aside, and jams the respirator hose back onto my neck. My lungs fill with air. My chest expands. I'm saved! I survive!

"You should turn the alarm off when you suction," the young man tells Pearl. Jesus Christ, if the alarm had been off he wouldn't have known anything was wrong. I'd be dead.

"Just give me a call if you need any help. I'm working down the hall," he says after suctioning me and giving her another lesson. Pearl nods vaguely. Guess he's a nurse. I don't know.

This can't last forever. There will be an end. Remember, Mexico in February. I see it all clearly. Rikki and I are at our favorite hotel in Puerto Vallarta. The visit with my parents is over. We're alone. We have breakfast under a cool canopy of palms on a patio overlooking the Pacific. A lazy day stretches ahead. What to do? Should we stay at the hotel, go sailing or rent a jeep. No pressure. Doesn't matter.

I'll be completely recovered by then. Hope I won't limp or use a cane. This will all be behind us—something to forget. Evenings, drinks in hand, we'll watch spectacular sunsets. Relaxing from relaxing.

I have the splints on. They're okay on my hands but

they cut into my feet. If Charlie saw that, he'd loosen them. Jesus, I hate this, hate Pearl. She's so fucking dumb.

I'm frightened and confused. People are suddenly crowding my room, even spilling out into the hall. Where did they come from? There's a striking looking black man with a Caribbean accent and several other people. Now I understand. They're here to weigh me.

Thank God they've ripped the splints off. Don't want those weighed. They're pushing in a massive steel scale. How are they going to get me on that metal slab? Oh, Jesus, they're lifting me. Please don't drop me, please.

"Hey Al, how much you figure this one weighs?" asks the Caribbean accent. Al guesses about 190. Someone else says 185. "You crazy man?" asks Al. "This here is a fat boy. Maybe over 200 pounds." I weighed less than 195 when I first got sick. They must be over feeding me!

They have me on the scale now. I'm lying on cold, hard steel and something sharp is digging into my right shoulder. Please hurry. My hospital gown is up around my chest. I'm completely exposed. Don't they know there is a person who feels inside this body?

They're laughing, making fun of me. What if I were grossly fat. If I weighed 300 pounds they'd be hysterical with laughter, rolling on the floor, pounding their fists with glee. Jesus, what's slicing into my shoulder? One of the splints must be stuck to me. The hard plastic is digging into me.

Hurry, you fucking bastards, hurry! Caribbean Al is moving the weights. "Don't cheat, mother fucker," someone warns him.

"I was right, man," he tells them with his musical accent. This is one big mother. Two-hundred-and-four pounds!" There's another eruption of laughter.

"He's big. Should have bet my money on him."

Shit. Stop talking and move me. Get me off this fucking slab. Get the splint out of my shoulder. They're lifting -- up high again, scared, scared, scared! Sons-of-bitches don't drop me! Jesus, safe on the bed, on my right side, on that same shoulder. Pain's still there. Splint must still be stuck to me. Oh, Jesus!

They're leaving. They're rolling the scale out of the room. I'm flashing Pearl. Get this fucking thing out of me!

"What's wrong?" she asks. How can I tell you what's wrong? Just look and find out! I swing my eyes back and forth so violently that the room spins. I'm on a carousel. "I know something is bothering you." Yes! Yes! "What's wrong? What is it?" She's trying to understand. She is concerned. It could be worse. She could be ignoring me.

Finally, she sees the splint, lifts my shoulder and pulls it out. "You poor, dear," she says. "That must have really hurt." It's her first words that show any kindness or warmth. I flash her a yes.

It's late, but there is no end to this day. Dr. Fittipaldi, a man in his early thirties, and his assistant, a sexy brunette, have arrived. Are they on the night shift? Dr. Fittipaldi strongly resembles Colonel Muammar el-Qaddafi, the Libyan dictator. Like Qaddafi, he's big and handsome and has wild curly hair, dark skin and mesmerizing eyes. He gives me a quick examination.

"This thing really wiped you out," he says with a sympathetic sigh of wonderment. He'll start the plasmapheresis as soon as they can get it scheduled, he promises. He'll be back another time to talk to Rikki and have her sign some forms.

They're about to leave. He suddenly stops and faces me. He must know he's a double for Qaddafi. "Arise," he orders, stretching his arms over his head. "I command you to rise." I'd laugh if I could. He's funny as hell.

I hear him chatting with his assistant as they go down the corridor. They're a great looking couple. Wonder if they're lovers. Be natural to walk with them, join their conversation. Can't walk or talk with anyone. Wonder if Dr. Fittipaldi, after seeing someone like me, ever realizes how lucky he is. Do beautiful people reflect?

"Time to catheterize you," says Pearl.

Oh, Jesus, she'll hurt me badly with this! The doctors removed my catheter a couple of days ago. To leave it in longer would risk infection. So now a nurse catheterizes me three or four times a day, each time sliding a tube up through my penis to my bladder. Somehow it hasn't hurt me.

Pearl rips open the box. It has lubricant, gloves, and the tube with a bag on its end to collect the urine. Almost everything's plastic: the box, the tube, the bag. What did hospitals do before plastic?

She's fooling around with my penis. Jesus, somehow she's managed it without hurting me. It must be the easiest thing in the world to do. Can't get over it. Has to be a piece of cake.

"I'm going to dinner now," Pearl says. What do you mean? You can't leave me! You're my nurse. You're supposed to take care of me. You can't go! I haven't been completely alone since I've been sick.

At Nyack I was in an open ward. Other nurses could see me. Here I'm in a room, out of view. At Nyack I was wired with sensors that sounded alarms if anything was wrong. The only alarm I have now is in the respirator. What happens if my heart stops? Will anyone know? Will anyone care?

Pearl's gone. There was no way I could stop her. So far so good. Don't need suctioning. I could be turned. I could always be turned. So tired. I'm so tired. There's less light in the corridor now. Don't know what time it is. Must be getting late.

Someone is calling my name. I feel I'm in a dream, but I'm wide-awake. "Robert Samuels! There's a phone call for Robert Samuels!" Sure, I'll take it. Tell them to hold on while I jump out of bed.

"Which one is Samuels?" asks the man calling my name.

"That one in there."

"Oh, guess he can't come to the phone." I hear him walking back down the hall.

What will he tell the caller? Will he simply say I'm not available, or will he lay on a shot of brutal reality: Samuels is unable to speak to you. In fact, he's unable to speak at all. He's mute. There's a tube in his neck connecting him to a machine. He can't breathe without the machine. He can't do many, many things. Like what, you ask. Well, he can't walk, or laugh, or smile, or blink, or scratch his nose. I doubt if he could even fart if he had to. He can weep and does.

Wish they'd come and tell me who was on the phone. It was probably some friend who couldn't believe that I'm paralyzed. I can't believe it myself. Rikki says everyone is calling to ask about me. She's sick of talking about it so Marilyn takes most of the calls. Marilyn is good on the phone. She asks if they want to call back and leave a message for me on tape.

The secretions are building. Soon I'll need suctioning. What happens then? How did I ever wind up with Pearl? How could this hospital send me someone like her? Why do we have to hire our own nurses? I thought this was the big time, the major leagues. Where's my room with a view?

Where the hell is Pearl! She must be having a five-course meal.

"How you doing?" asks the male nurse from down the hall. I swing my eyes back and forth to show him something's wrong. "Bet you need suctioning." Eyes right. He takes care of it quickly and easily.

Pearl is back. "Just suctioned your patient," he tells her. She nods dully.

We're alone. I swing my eyes. Turn me. You haven't turned me. She doesn't notice. My pillows are rock hard. Now the terrible sweats are upon me. I always count on those to save me. She'll see me awash and that will force her to turn me. I sweat and sweat unnoticed.

"Time for your dinner," she says, getting up to start the white stuff flowing to my nose. Don't you see how wet I am? Turn me now!

The white stuff has finished flowing through the feeding tube and she still hasn't turned me. To clean the tube, she runs water through it. The dirty-looking water goes right to my stomach. I guess there's nothing wrong with this since all the nurses do it, but I feel like I'm drinking dishwater.

She detaches the long tube from my short nose tube. The nose tube must give me the look of an elephant. I'm the size of an elephant. Can't believe I weigh 204. They stuffed me at Nyack, constantly poured the white stuff into me. Have to diet again when I get out of here.

Can't stand this any longer. The terrible sweats have stopped and still she hasn't turned me. TURN ME NOW, YOU FUCKING BITCH! She turns me. Total bliss! It's as good as an orgasm. Fuck the bath; fuck everything. I'm off that side. Now I face the wall.

Pearl is telling a woman with a black southern accent about me. Who is she? Can't see. Don't hear them now. There's a sound. Someone in the room. "Let me look at you, darling," says the woman. I'm being turned. Black face. Middle-aged woman in nurse's uniform. "I'm Ida," she says, "your night nurse."

No smile but that's okay—that's friendly enough for me. Already she's talked more than Pearl did during her entire shift. "You look damp," she says, feeling my chest with a rough, calloused hand. "You been sweatin'?" I flash a yes. "Now why didn't Pearl give you a bath if you been sweatin' like that?" I don't know. Beats me.

"I don't mind giving you a bath. I don't mind doing nothing if it happens on my time. That's my job. Just don't like doing something not on my time, you understand?" Yes.

Suddenly she seems to attack me. She rips off the sheet, and then jerks my arm through the hospital gown. She scrubs me as if I have baked-on grease. She rolls me this way and that. My arm twists under me; my face hits the guardrail. My eyes tear with the pain. I need suctioning. She stabs my throat, mouth, and nostrils with the catheter.

Now she's changing the sheets. I roll, my face again slamming into the guardrail. What does it take to break a nose? She's shoving the bed away from the wall to roll me back the other way, my face banging into the other guardrail. Is she doing this because she's pissed at Pearl or is this just her usual style?

The assault is over. I'm on my side, facing the wall again. Lights off. She sits. Silence. The only sound is the respirator. Darkness. She can't see my eyes if I need help. Fuck her. I don't want her to see me.

Try to move. Maybe Dr. Schwartz was right. Maybe I can move if I really try. Try, really try, you stupid bastard. No way. Nothing doing. The circuits are down. A hurricane took out my lines. Maybe she's turned off the lights because she expects me to sleep. That's reasonable. It is night. Most people sleep at night but I know I won't sleep.

Rikki's alone in our bed. Hope she's asleep. Must be lonely, even with Marilyn in the house. Wonder if Rikki stays on her side of the bed or uses it all when I'm not there. Never thought to ask.

I remember sleeping alone in that bed only once. It was five or six years ago when Charlie was away and Rikki was in the hospital. Except for Ruffy and Sam, our unfriendly cat, the house was empty. Rikki was scheduled that morning for a tubal ligation, a cutting of her fallopian tubes with a laser, to keep her from getting pregnant. Her gynecologist thought if she stopped using the loop for birth control, it might ease her menstrual cramps.

When Rikki had asked what I thought of the doctor's suggestion, I'd acted like a pompous ass. "It's your body and you have to decide if you'll ever want more children," I'd told her. Where did I get that line? A half-hour later she called the doctor and told him she wanted to go ahead.

Before I knew it, she was in New York Hospital and I was alone in the bed. It was happening so quickly because Rikki wanted to be completely well before we left on vacation.

In that empty bed, I suddenly became very frightened. What if she died from the anesthesia or the operation? Had we decided too quickly? No second opinions. I copped out. It's your decision, darling. Bullshit! The dearest person in the world to me and I'm careless with her life. It was a long, long night.

I drove to work that day—Texaco's offices were still in the city—and, coming down the East River Drive, I passed Rikki's hospital. It was all I could do to make myself go on. I wanted to burst in and call it off. Live with the menstrual cramps!

I kept going, didn't stop. I spent some nervous hours at work before telling Warren what was bothering me. He sat talking with me until, at last, the phone rang. Rikki was fine. My luck was very good that day.

Is Ida sleeping? What time is it now? There's a window in this room so I'll know when dawn comes. But remember, December has the longest nights.

Lights on. Ida's checking the respirator, checking me. Not bad. If only she weren't so rough. Maybe she'll turn me. I'm flashing my eyes. "What do you want? You want to be turned?" Yes, yes. Slam, bang, face into the guardrail. Jesus, this woman is insane. She can't still be angry at Pearl, can she?

Lights off again. This time I'm facing away from the wall. I see Ida through the darkness. She sits erect, not sleeping. What next? I watch.

~

She's up giving me eye drops, then lights out once more. As time passes, she catheterizes, feeds, suctions, and turns me. She takes my temperature, pulse and blood pressure. She beats my chest to loosen the congestion. She slams my face into the guardrail each time she turns me. I am afraid of her.

Ida's on her break and I lie here worried. I know when she returns she'll see that I'm into the terrible sweats and she'll bathe me, change the sheets, and brutalize me.

She's back now, bouncing my face off the rails. Has she loosened the capped tooth in the front of my mouth? I can't move my tongue to feel it. Hope she's bruised my face. People will notice. They'll fire her.

I'm facing the wall. Dim, grey light filters through my sooty window. After the dawn Rikki will come. I will wait until then. I will not move my eyes to beg Ida for help. Although my pillows are stone, I will endure. Rikki will turn me gently. I adore her. I hear someone. It's not Ida or Rikki. Rikki would speak. I move my eyes, shift them left and right, to attract attention.

It's a new nurse. "I was hoping you wouldn't see me until after I got my makeup on," she says.

She leans over to look at me. "You want to be turned?" she guesses. Yes. You're brilliant!

"Okay," she sighs, "I'll turn you." Thank you. Now I'm facing the room. She's putting on makeup at the sink near the door—the room has no bathroom. She's strikingly pretty and buxom, nice hips. Sexy. Skinny isn't the only look.

Rikki's here. She slides gracefully around the nurse into the room. She sees only me. "Are you okay, darling?" she asks. Yes. "Was your night all right?" Yes. I don't want her to know about the rails.

"I'm Ingrid Carpenter," says the new nurse. "You're Mrs. Samuels?"

"That's right," replies Rikki. "I'm Bob's wife. Why don't you call me Rikki?"

Ingrid Carpenter is intelligent, articulate and very immature. She's an Army brat, daughter of an officer. She grew up on bases all over the United States and Europe. Her parents now live in Washington D.C.

"My father's a domineering bastard and my mother is a sniveling weakling," she tells us vehemently. Who asked?

She began nursing here after graduating from Columbia. Since then she's become a nursing bum, working in various New York hospitals, and hospitals in the Washington area. Why Washington if she hates her parents, I wonder.

She's never been married. There have been lovers, of course. There's no one serious right now, but she has a continuing relationship with a "brilliant" doctor who is married and practices in Boston. "We hope to be together over Christmas," she announces defiantly.

We are to understand that she's not just another nurse. She's unique and *in-ter-est-ing*!

"All I own is my car—a Honda," she boasts. "I don't even have my own apartment. I live with a girl friend on West End Avenue but she's getting sick of me and I'm fed up with her. I want to get out of the city. I want to live some place where there's grass and trees. I'm tired of stepping over garbage and dog shit."

She's in her mid-thirties, I'd guess, an overage, half-assed hippie. Life's a disappointment. Nothing ever lives up to her expectations. In the suburbs she'd be complaining of the dull sameness of everything.

When she tries, she's not a bad nurse, but most of the time she's distracted and sloppy. She puts nothing back in place so my small room is soon a mess. She's also very lazy.

Rikki desperately wants to help take care of me. She cheerfully picks up after Ingrid, suggesting places to store things. Ingrid's agreeable—she's more than willing to have someone do her work and listen to her stories and complaints.

"I like her," Rikki says when Ingrid goes to have a cigarette. "Do you?" Yes, I lie.

"She seems to be a good nurse." Yes, I agree, she has her good points. She's not brutal, not dangerously ignorant.

Ordinarily, Rikki would find Ingrid impossibly immature and neurotic. Now she clings to her. There's no one else. Pearl is so creepy but Ingrid at least is a familiar middle-class type. Rikki wants to trust someone; she needs to trust someone.

Before the morning is out, they're talking like old friends. Together they bathe me. Then it's time for chest physical therapy. They roll me on my side. Ingrid beats my ribs to demonstrate, and then Rikki tries. "Harder," Ingrid tells her, and Rikki pounds me harder.

"You sure I'm not hurting Bob?" Rikki asks. "No, that doesn't hurt," Ingrid assures her. Ingrid's wrong.

"Am I hurting you?" Rikki asks me. No, I tell her. The truth would bring her to tears.

Dr. Ramsbotham enters, wearing a bright orange tie and pushing a machine covered with dials and trailing wires. He and his machine crowd the room. The machine reminds me of the one that shocked the Frankenstein monster to life. I hope it does something similar for me.

"How are you today, sir?" Dr. Ramsbotham asks politely. I flash him a yes. "What's he saying?" he asks Rikki.

"That means yes. Eyes to the right means yes."

"Well, yes. That's very good. I brought my portable EMG machine. I'd like to do a test on your nerves later. Is that all right, sir?" Yes. You're my doctor. Do what you think best.

"What's he saying?"

"He's saying yes," Rikki answers patiently, "and please call him Bob, not he," she adds.

Suddenly, I need suctioning. Dr. Ramsbotham doesn't want to watch. He flees, shouting a warning back through the doorway about not touching the machine. It costs $10,000, he says. That's not much for medical equipment, Ingrid points out when he's gone.

Ingrid is at lunch. Rikki is pumping my legs as we listen to the tape of the calls. There are too many to keep track of. "Are you glad we made the move?" Rikki asks. Yes. Despite the problems with nurses, despite the crummy room, we did the right thing.

Time is passing. They've taken the day's second set of chest x-rays. Hope Dr. Schick is reading them, not letting me drown. I can't tell how I'm doing. It doesn't seem difficult to breathe but the respirator, or ventilator as Dr. Schick calls it, is doing all the work. It won't keep me from dying if the sacs in my lungs fill with fluids, blocking the oxygen.

Dr. Ramsbotham has returned for the EMG test. He begins by putting what he says is a contact device on my arm and painlessly inserting small needles in my hand. He's very exact in placing the needles. In professorial tones, he explains how he'll now send charges through my nerves to test how well they conduct electricity. The more current they carry the better, is my understanding. When he's satisfied that everything's set, he starts the machine. Zap, zap, zap. The first zaps are barely perceptible. Then he slowly increases the power and the zaps become jolts. The pain is agonizing.

I hate this test but I endure it. After all, it's for my own good. It can't last forever. Zap, zap, zap, ZAP! JOLT! JOLT! JOLT! "Just a few more, sir." I brace myself. The anticipation is worse than the pain. JOLT! JOLT! JOLT! He's moving the needles.

He reads the results on dials and paper scroll that curls slowly out of the machine. Dr. Ramsbotham reports he's getting almost no readings from my nerves. My insulation is stripped away. Rikki watches, not knowing what I'm suffering. If she knew, she'd demand he stop the test. I can't let her do that.

Dr. Ramsbotham is incredibly polite. He seems embarrassed by the pain he's inflicting. "Not long now, sir," he promises after dozens of shocks. JOLT! JOLT! He's been at it maybe a half-hour. "There, that will do. That's enough, sir. There's been quite substantial damage to the myelin, he says.

"I've finished the right side of your body. We'll do the left side another time." You mean you've only done half? I'll have to go through this again? Do you think the left side will be different?

"Has Bob reached a plateau," Rikki asks him.

"I don't know, but one would assume he has."

"How long will it take for him to recover?"

"It's difficult to tell now," he says. "Let's see what affect plasmapheresis has, but I would start thinking of his recovery in terms of weeks, not days." Weeks, I think, weeks! I have so many more miles to go before I sleep, so many more days before I'm home.

"Good day, sir" he tells me, pushing his machine, with its dangling wires, awkwardly out the door.

"Did you hear him, darling?" asks Rikki, clutching my hand. "He says he thinks you've reached the plateau. You're starting to recover. Isn't that great news?" I flash her a yes, but I'm numb. Weeks, not days, weeks!

Dale and Stanley, who arrived simultaneously, have taken Rikki out for coffee. That's just as well since Dr. Schick is here to check my lungs. She's using a stethoscope with two cold metal disks instead of the usual one. She must be listening in stereo. There won't be a bronchoscopy today, she says. The chest p.t. has done some good. My lungs are beginning to hold their own. I'm excited. Rikki is right—things are beginning to improve. Why hadn't they tried chest p.t. at Nyack?

"I'm unhappy about your weight. You're too fat." Dr. Schick says. Before I go spinning off into my usual depression about my weight she adds, "If you're heavy, it will be harder for you to hold yourself up between the parallel bars when you start walking."

Walking! She's actually talking about me walking! I'll be better soon! Maybe days, not weeks. If Rikki could only hear this. I wish there were some way for me to tell her when she gets back.

Dr. Schick is lousy at math. She needs Ingrid's help to calculate my proper caloric intake. Ingrid is like a kid eager to show the teacher how bright she is. I'm no common nurse—I'm a fascinating person!

In the midst of the calculations, Pearl arrives to relieve Ingrid. "You did a great job with the chest p.t.," Dr. Schick tells her. The praise means nothing to Pearl, but Ingrid's face flushes with jealousy. Rikki's return crowds the room. Good thing Dr. Ramsbotham took his machine with him. Rikki is in a hurry because Stanley is waiting to walk her to our car. Before I know it, she's out the door and gone. No one told her the good news about me walking.

Now Ingrid is gone too. Only Pearl remains. The room is strangely quiet. There are tears in my eyes and desolation in my heart. I feel abandoned. There's no one here who knows me. I am Blanche Dubois, depending on the kindness of strangers. But unlike Blanche, I recite no brilliant Tennessee Williams lines. I am mute.

Outside it's dark. I picture the cold and dirty streets. My family lived just four blocks from this bed. For all I know, Rikki is parked in front of our old apartment house. This was where we were living when my mother died.

She died during surgery for stomach cancer when I was five. Her death crushed my father. In his grief, he clung to the idea that my sister and I should remain with him. We were a family. He didn't want us living with relatives.

There were no maiden aunts available to move in with us, so he hired a housekeeper, actually, as it turned out, a series of housekeepers, other peoples' maiden aunts. They were quite a bunch. One trembled and cried every time he spoke to her, one drank and one wanted to marry him. (He told me once that he had been so desperately lonely that he almost had married her but he knew he'd regret it because she wasn't very bright.) And there was Auntie Cline. I loved her.

She probably wasn't more than forty-five, but when I think of her now, I see a very old woman wearing black dresses. She was a "licensed practical nurse." I'd hear my father tell family and friends, "The children are being cared for by a licensed practical nurse." I was very impressed by that and apparently he was too.

Auntie Cline was also a practicing Roman Catholic. I am descended, on both sides, from long lines of non-practicing, non-religious Jews. We celebrated Christmas—which also happens to be my birthday—as an American holiday. Christmas meant a Christmas tree and Santa Claus, not the birth of Jesus. Easter was colored eggs and chocolate bunnies, nothing more.

We are Jews ethnically, not religiously. My father said they had persecuted our people for 2,000 years and right now the Nazis were sending Jews to death camps in Europe. To deny we were Jews would be shameful. I had only the haziest idea of what he was talking about but if he thought it important to be Jewish, I was glad I was.

Auntie Cline moved quickly to fill what she saw as my religious vacuum. I was soon accompanying her to Mass. Our visits seemed unplanned. We'd drop by the church while shopping or doing an errand. My sister, who was ten or eleven, never came with us.

I didn't like the musty gloom of the local parish church or the odd smell of incense. The Latin services were incomprehensible and boring but Auntie Cline told me how God was good and how you could talk to Him by praying. I imagined my folded hands were my microphone to Him— my own little radio transmitter to heaven.

I'd wait when Auntie Cline made her confession. The carved, wooden booths seemed to me a wonderful place for telling secrets. Someday, Auntie Cline promised, I would be allowed to sit in one and make my own confession. She gave me my very own rosary beads. That was her undoing.

One evening, after Auntie Cline had tucked me in, my father came into my room to say good night. As he sat on the side of my bed talking, his hand slid under my pillow. "What's this?" he demanded, pulling out the beads.

"It's my rosary." I proudly told him.

Auntie Cline was gone by the time I got up the next morning. Soon after, my father gave up trying to keep us with him. My sister and I moved to his parents' house in Ozone Park, Queens. We lived there until my father married Louise several years later.

Pearl is going to kill me! When she suctions, she disconnects the respirator long before she needs to. Doesn't she realize I can't breathe without it?

People have rushed in here three times tonight because my respirator keeps beeping. They think it's an emergency, that I'm unattended and that the hose between the machine and my neck has somehow disconnected. When they see Pearl is with me, they are relieved. Don't they understand that she's incompetent? They must not want to get involved. But maybe I overestimate the danger. Maybe that's why they do nothing.

Caribbean, one of the attendants who weighed me, is here. Even though he made fun of me, it's impossible to stay angry with him. He's a charming, beautiful man with shiny black skin and a dazzling white smile. "How you feeling, man?" I flash him a yes.

"You making it man?" Yes.

"You ever been in Trinidad?" Yes. I am lying. I never lie about my travels, but I so much want his guy to like me.

"You like Trinidad?" Yes.

"Beautiful island, man?" Yes. Oh what a tangled web we weave...

"You be better for Christmas," he declares. It's not a question; it's a flat statement. He's saying I'll be better by Christmas. I have a friend. Now I'm glad I lied.

Pearl is standing back against the wall. Her skin is pale café au lait. Caribbean is polished ebony. He's so vital and she's so wan. Suddenly he bursts into song: "I'll be home for Christmas...." Look out Harry Belafonte!

Ida is here to start work. I made it through Pearl's shift— cheated death again. Ida's a much better nurse than Pearl. Her only terrible fault is her roughness. That can't kill me. If she breaks my nose, it will be painful but I'll survive.

This time I won't let her hurt me. I will avoid having her turn me. It is better to lie here aching from discomfort than to be slammed into the rails like a hockey player into the boards. I am determined. I will not ask her to turn me.

Ida sits in the dark. I lie staring. How much time has passed? The next time she checks something, I will signal her to turn me. I am weak. I wait for the light. Nothing to do but wait. Face it, the bitch is never going to turn on the light. Perhaps she's done everything she has to do for the night. Has she? Has she catheterized me, fed me, taken my vital signs, bathed me? Jesus, I can't remember what she's done. I don't think she's bathed me.

Will you ever turn on the light? How can you sit here in the dark like this, you fucking moron? I couldn't do it. If I'm waiting, I need something to read. People get on airplanes, heading out across the Pacific, without a book or even a magazine. Nearly twenty hours of staring at nothing. Amazing! I can't even sit on a toilet without literature. How many times have I read the back of a tube of Crest?

I shift my eyes but it does no good. She can't see me in the dark. She's not a cat, although she sits as quietly as one. What if she's dead? People do die. This morning Ingrid will find a living patient and a dead nurse. It will make a great headline for the New York Post: Dead Nurse Tends Critically Ill Patient. Move me now you stupid bitch, I scream silently.

Could she have heard me? She's up and the light is on. She has the towels, the basin, and the Ivory soap. The way she scrubs, she should be using Comet and Brillo. Does she think I'm a dirty frying pan? I don't care. To have her turn me is worth the price in pain.

Here it comes! She's rolling me. Ah, the relief! God, I love it. No, no! I'm going too fast. My face is into the railing, my eyes tear from the sharp pain. Christ my arm, my shoulder too is caught, twisted painfully under me. It feels dislocated. Oh, shit it hurts! It wasn't worth the price. I shouldn't have been weak and wanted her to turn me.

It's daylight now. Ida is muttering about Ingrid. "I have to move my car. If she doesn't come soon, I'll get a ticket." Good. I hope they tow your car away and dump it in the river.

Rikki's here. "How are you this morning, darling," she says, bending to kiss me. Yes, I flash. She's come early to meet Ida, to let Ida know I'm human, that I have a wife and family who loves me. As if Ida would give a shit.

At the beginning of each school year, Rikki would insist on meeting Charlie's teachers. She wanted them to understand that he had a mother who cared, who thought him special. She's using the same tactic to help me. It's not working because Ida is thinking only about the parking ticket she might get if Ingrid doesn't show up soon. That's all she cares about.

Ingrid finally breezes in. She's full of fake-sounding excuses for being late, but before she can finish giving them, Ida's out the door, racing the cops to her car. Hope she loses.

Ingrid drives me crazy. She talks incessantly and when she talks, she stops all other motion. This leads to absurd situations. For example, I'll be lying here ready to be catheterized, nightgown pulled up, private parts completely aired, and she'll start yakking, making vague philosophic points about the sad state of American medicine. Meanwhile, I'm left exposed, like some crazy man on the subway. Suddenly, she'll pause mid-sentence and ask Rikki to remind her what she was about to do. "I think you were catheterizing Bob."

"Oh yes," she says, finally giving me her full attention. Glad she's not a brain surgeon.

It's afternoon. Rikki has been gone hours, trying to iron out problems about paying the nurses. I have good medical coverage and we'll probably be reimbursed later, but no one knows how much later. She's writing checks as if our account were a bottomless pit. It's a massive cash flow problem. Rikki is frantic with worry.

Dr. Fittipaldi, the Qaddafi look-alike, is here without his gorgeous assistant. He wants Rikki to sign the forms giving permission for the plasmapheresis. Ingrid asks him to wait a few minutes for Rikki's return.

Even without my glasses, I can see he turns Ingrid on. She's ready to hop in the sack with him. All it would take is for him to nod, to wink. I have visions of them embracing, his hand sliding up under her white skirt. They fall entangled on top of me, writhing, panting. Watch the respirator hose, please.

Rikki has returned, completely overwrought from her experiences at the nurses' registry. She willingly signs the consent forms, asking when the treatments will begin. Soon, Dr. Fittipaldi promises. The results could be dramatic, he adds, but on the other hand, it's all experimental. You can't be sure that it will do any good at all. There is no danger, however, he assures her.

Once more he goes into his act. Standing at the foot of my bed, he lifts his arms towards heaven. "Rise," he intones, "I command you to rise."

"You think this is a joke!" screams Rikki, shattering the room's convivial atmosphere. "This isn't funny. Are you a fool?" She's hysterical.

Dr. Fittipaldi stares at her as if she's a madwoman. "I don't have to take this!" he shouts. "I don't have to treat this man," he adds, stalking out.

Run after him, I want to say. Plead with him. Tell him you're sorry. Tell him you're upset.

"He's crazy," Rikki says. "There's no reason to put up with his crap." Yes there is. He's the only reason we're here. I need plasmapheresis. It's my only hope.

"What was he doing?" she asks Ingrid. "What was his point? Is he crazy?" she demands.

"I think he was making a joke." Ingrid tells her.

"A joke? My husband is completely paralyzed and he thinks it's funny." She looks at me. "I was right wasn't I?"

I swing my eyes to the right, then to the left. Even though I thought he was hilarious, I understand why you're upset. You think he's not taking our situation seriously. Then, to compound what he did, he walked out, threatening not to treat me. That was terrible. But it doesn't matter that you're right. I need him. He doesn't need us.

Although Ingrid's natural inclination is to foment trouble, she's trying to calm Rikki. Finally, she talks Rikki into writing Dr. Fittipaldi a note apologizing for her outburst.

It is mid-afternoon of another day. I've survived Pearl and Ida again. Dr Rossi, the beautiful Italian resident, has come to do a spinal tap. Oh Christ, please don't try sitting me up on the side of the bed. They have sent Rikki somewhere to wait.

"Bob," Dr. Rossi explains, "you don't have to let me do this, but you should know I think it's important. It will confirm that you have Guillain-Barré syndrome. Can I go ahead?"

Of course go ahead. Dr. Schwartz never did the second spinal tap at Nyack. Maybe I don't have Guillain-Barré. I want to know. Go ahead and tap my spine.

They don't try to sit me up. Dr. Rossi instead helps Ingrid bend me into a fetal position. Some men would hate being so powerless before women. It doesn't bother me at all. I prefer having a woman examine me. I don't understand why any guy wouldn't rather a woman touched him.

"Is your back numb?" Dr. Rossi asks rubbing it. Yes, I flash. I feel Ingrid's strong hands against my neck, pushing my head to bend my spine more. Now there's the intense pressure of Dr. Rossi pressing on the small of my back.

"It's in," she says with relief. My stomach churns sickeningly as she draws the fluid out.

Oh, I hate this so. Why don't all you bastards just go and leave me alone.

They're putting a bandage on the small of my back. Is it to stop my spinal fluid from leaking? Could it just dribble away? If it was happening, could I feel it and warn them? Could it be fatal? And why did they have to try to sit me up at Nyack to do this? I don't know. I just don't know anything.

Rikki has left for the day. It's Pearl's shift now. Dr. Ramsbotham stops in. "How are you today, sir?" he asks. I flash a yes. What does he think I would I say if I could talk? Does he imagine I'd tell him things are great?

"Oh, dear," he says. "What does he mean? I'm not very good at this."

"I don't know," replies Pearl.

"Can you move your feet?" he asks. His question couldn't astonish me more if he asked me to try to tap dance. It's my understanding that you start to recover from Guillain-Barré at your trunk and it works its way out to your extremities. My feet should be the last part of me that I can move.

Nevertheless, I try to move them. If an eminent expert on human flight said I should attempt to fly, I'd flap my arms and give it a shot. He might know something I don't. Maybe the spinal tap proved I don't have Guillain-Barré.

"That's all right, sir," Dr. Ramsbotham, tells me reassuringly when my feet don't budge. "The lumbar puncture shows the level of protein in the fluid to be quite high. It confirms the diagnosis made at Nyack.

"Is he triggering the respirator?" he asks Pearl as he watches my chest gently heave in response to the machine.

"Once in a while," she replies.

"Really, really!" he says, excited by the news. I hope it's something significant.

As far as I can tell, I haven't slept a moment in the nearly two weeks I've been sick. For the past couple of nights, I've been trying to bore myself to sleep and it's not working. Don't know why. God knows I'm dull enough.

It took me almost four years to live through the Air Force, and now it seems to be taking almost that long to relive it in my mind. I'm conjuring up obscure little facts I thought I'd long forgotten.

I'm now remembering my favorite assignment, at Hamilton Air Force Base in California, near San Francisco. I worked for a Sergeant Bisbee. My friend, Matt Baigell, and I hung out at a North Beach cafe, The Anxious Asp. We were fledgling writers searching for the beat generation. We never realized all those people had gone back to New York. We were a couple of years too late.

I can't stand doing this anymore! It's too fucking boring and it's not working—I'm still awake. I quit! Fuck it! My enlistment is not even half over but I'm giving myself an honorable discharge.

Dr. Schick is openly skeptical of Pearl's report of me triggering the respirator when she examines me. To do that, she explains, you have to breathe against it, resist it. A light would flash if this were happening, adds her assistant. There have been no flashing lights. I haven't triggered the respirator during her shifts, Ingrid assures them.

"It would be lovely if this were happening," Dr. Schick tells me, "but I'm afraid we won't see it for a while."

"Pearl doesn't know much about respirators," Ingrid comments, trying to let Dr. Schick know that she's the far superior nurse.

"She certainly doesn't," agrees Dr. Schick. Then why do you let Pearl take care of me, I want to scream. Aren't you risking my life?

Ingrid has told me that everyone considers Dr. Schick one of the hospital's real stars. I want to trust all these medical people, but they constantly give me reason to doubt. Dr. Schick, for example, agrees that Pearl is inadequate but acts as if it is unimportant. Why doesn't she do something about it? Pearl could kill me! Maybe I exaggerate.

Dr. Ramsbotham isn't much for day-to-day patient management (as they call it), so Dr. Schick has unofficially taken on most of what should be his responsibilities. Why is Dr. Ramsbotham so inadequate? Is he really a Guillain-Barré expert?

Pearl drifts in like a ghost. Ingrid's shift is over. Dr. Schick wants my feeding tube changed and moved from my right to left nostril. A tube shouldn't remain in one nostril too long, she says, and one of a narrower gauge might cut down my secretions. She's leaving orders about it in my chart, and tells Pearl that Ida should change the tube. I don't think Dr. Schick trusts Pearl to do it.

That was many hours ago. Ida's shift is almost over and she's done nothing about the nose tube. I'm hoping they lost the orders. Morning is almost here. The orders must have gotten screwed up. We've completed my daily scouring. Ida's dusting me with powder. She's the only one that uses it. I can't stand the damn powder.

"Got to change your nose tube," she says unexpectedly. I'm startled. She almost never talks.

She cranks up the back of the bed. The equipment here is so ancient that the nurses literally have to turn a handle to raise or lower parts of the bed. Why doesn't this world-famous hospital have electric beds?

I'm scared. She has me in a semi-sitting position. My head is slumped on my chest. I stare at the fresh sheet covering my stomach. It seems so strange. I haven't sat up or seen my body in days and days.

Before I can worry about how much removing the tube will hurt, she's tugging at it. It's coming out! It doesn't hurt, but it releases a fresh eruption of mucus. It's as if the tube had blocked everything. Now Ida's roughly jamming the suction catheter into my mouth and nose. I'm a human being, you bitch!

Oh Jesus, she has the new nose tube in her hand and she's forcing it up one nostril. It doesn't go. She keeps stabbing it in my nose. It hurts like crazy and makes my eyes tear. I see the tears raining down on the crisp, white sheet.

"I don't know how to do this," she admits. You're telling me, I want to say. "I'm going to leave it for the day nurse. You'll have to skip your breakfast today. We can't feed you until they get the tube in." Hooray, hooray! I don't give a fuck about breakfast.

I'm happy now because Rikki is here. We're waiting for Ingrid. I love this time alone with Rikki, without nurses. She sits holding my hand, telling me about everything that's happening at home. Someone still loves me, remembers I'm me.

Rikki's been coming in before eight every morning so that Ida can leave on time. Otherwise, Ida would have to wait and risk a parking ticket. Ingrid is always 15 minutes to 30 minutes late.

We're in a trap, paying a hundred dollars a shift for these nurses. How did we assemble such a crew? Pearl is dangerously incompetent. Ida is brutal. And Ingrid, the best of the lot, is a neurotic, man-hungry, immature slob. Does anyone screen these women? Does the hospital take any responsibility for seeing that they are qualified?

Ingrid is flustered today about being late, as though it's something unusual. She barely has her coat off and she's asking, "Where's his nose tube?" Rikki doesn't know. She hadn't even realized it was gone. I had completely forgotten about it. "There's no way to feed him," Ingrid says. "He'll starve!" At first I think she's kidding.

"Have you had your morning feeding?" she asks, making it sound like I'm an animal in a zoo. No, I flash. She's in a real panic. The excitement pleases me. It's something different to break up the routine.

"Are you worried?" Rikki asks after Ingrid is out of the room and down the hall, looking for help. No, I flash. I'm not.

Ingrid's quickly back. Dr. Rossi is off, she reports. The resident covering this floor today is busy. He's told Ingrid to try to put the nose tube in herself.

I'm sitting up again, head pitched down. Ingrid has a new tube. She's trying to push it up my right nostril. Drool slobbers from my mouth, to my chin and to the sheets, making big stains near the tiny dots my tears left earlier. Oh, dear God, end this!

Ingrid's pushing hard. There's a sharp pain and a ripping sound in my nose. Blood drips, making new spots on the sheets.

Oh, shit," Ingrid says, softly, "I'm sorry." She gently pushes my head back and holds tissues to my nose to stop the bleeding. She's very calm now. It is a situation that would panic most people. It's so strange. Only a few minutes ago she was hysterical over nothing.

I see Rikki. She's looking on helplessly, biting the side of her hand to keep from crying out. Her face is filled with pain and despair. I wish I could reach out and hold her in my arms. It's all right, my darling, I'd say. It's only a bloody nose.

We'll soon be on the beach in Mexico. At night I'll sleep holding you close. All this will soon be a memory.

I suddenly realize why the tube won't go up there. It is my deviated septum. The tissue between my two nostrils has always been bent, obstructing the right side. There's no way I can tell Ingrid.

She's trying my left nostril now, the one that had the tube. She has it part way up, but it backs up and coils in her hand. She doesn't panic. She keeps trying but it's not going in. Ignore the pain, I tell myself. It will soon be over.

"We'll have to get the resident," she tells us, giving up at last. She's leaving the room to call him. I can't tolerate sitting up any longer. I'm flashing at Rikki.

"What's wrong?" she pleads, "What's wrong?" She runs after Ingrid and pulls her back to the room.

"You want to be moved?" Ingrid guesses immediately. Yes, I flash. Move me now! Let me lie down!

"You have to stay in this position. The resident will want you sitting up." No, I flash. Fuck the resident! Fuck the tube! I have to lie down!

She ignores me. She's gone. I'm crying. Tears of rage are falling on the sheet, joining the other stains. Will this ever end?

Shit, fuck, I'm choking. The klaxon on the respirator is sounding. Vinnie rushes in. "Where's his nurse?" he demands, suctioning me furiously.

"Gone to get the resident," Rikki replies. "Bob needs a new nose tube."

"Oh," says Vinnie, finishing suctioning.

"Vinnie," asks Rikki, "before you go, could you move Bob?" Oh, sweet angel love of mine!

"Move him? Move him? What you mean move him?"

"Put him on his side. Let him lie down."

"I don't have time," Vinnie says. "Ask his regular nurse."
Fuck! Shit! Piss! Vinnie, you little bastard! You fuck!

Think of something else. Stare at the sheet. Notice the interesting mosaic the stains make. Think of that, not the agony of sitting up.

It is difficult to tell which stains are which, except for the blood. It's already turned brown. Those spots are like those on a virgin bride's sheets. Once I deflowered a virgin. Once is enough. Virgins, virgins, think of virgins. Each time a virgin passes, the lions in front of the New York Public Library roar, my father once told me. The lions are stone. Was Ingrid ever a virgin? Oh, where is fucking Ingrid!

"Should I try to move you?" Rikki asks desperately. No! You might disconnect the respirator. You might hurt me. No!

"Should I get Ingrid?" Yes!

"The doctor is coming soon," Ingrid tells us as she rushes back into the room.

"Bob wants to lie down," Rikki says.

"The doctor will want him sitting up."

"He wants to lie down now!" she repeats. Her voice is steel. Rikki, you're wonderful.

Ingrid yields. With each turn of the crank, I feel more relief. "It doesn't make any sense," she complains, "We'll only have to put him up again." Screw you, Ingrid!

The resident hasn't come. We've been waiting over a half an hour. Rikki is pumping my legs, my favorite activity. I know it's hard for Rikki. My heavy legs strain her back. We're listening to the tape of yesterday's phone calls. Warren updates me on office politics. Frank Dougherty, who works with me on the magazine, gives me the latest change in the printing schedule.

We're listening to the tape on an AM-FM cassette player I bought Charlie for his tenth birthday. I remember his

excitement when he got it. That doesn't seem so long ago.
Glad Charlie thought of having Rikki bring the tapes each
day. It's helped me from feeling totally isolated.

The resident is thin, hollowed-eyed and very nervous.
He hasn't slept or shaved for a while. He must be in his
twenties but he could be mistaken for twice that. I feel a
slight tremble in his hand as he holds my head. Do it! Get the
damn tube up my nose! Get it over!

"I talked with Dr. Schick and she wants a thinner tube
and she wants it in his right nostril," he tells Ingrid. It won't
go up the right nostril, asshole, I want to scream.

It starts again. He's pushing but the tube won't do what
he wants. Fuck this! Let me starve!

He tries over and over, but he's not getting it. Nothing's
working. My chin is on my chest. I'm again staring at the
spotted sheet. Drool, tears, and blood—more drips than a
Jackson Pollock painting. Bet Pollock never put this much of
himself in his work.

Fuck it! I'm flashing, shifting my eyes back and forth as
quickly as I can. I want out. I want to lie down. "What's he
want?" asks the resident.

"He wants to lie down," says Ingrid.

"I have to finish," he tells me "Then you can lie down."
When will that be? When the fuck will that be?

"I don't know why, but I can't get it in this nostril," he
says. "Something's blocking it." No shit, Dick Tracy.

He's trying the right nostril now. I feel it going in.

"I have it," he says, with relief. No, you don't, shithead!
It's curling in my mouth. The fucking tube is through my nose
and into my mouth, filling it like plastic spaghetti.

I'm flashing, trying to get his attention, let him know
things are wrong. "Bob, you can't lie down until we're done,"
says Ingrid. No, no, the fucking tube is in my mouth. I'm trying

to help you!

It's curling out between my lips. Ingrid sees it. "The tube is coming out of his mouth," she reports.

"Oh, shit," says the resident. He looks totally defeated. Quit! Go home. Go to sleep. I don't need food. Everyone says I'm too fat. "I need some help," the resident admits.

We wait for the next development. This time there's no argument about letting me lie down.

Ingrid is obviously pleased that someone else is having trouble with the tube, but she hasn't forgotten to blame Ida. "It was irresponsible of her to go off without telling us about the nose tube. There's no excuse for that. You should get rid of her," she declares, seizing a fresh opportunity to make trouble.

"I can't decide that," Rikki says. "She's Bob's nurse. Should I get rid of Ida?" she asks me.

At first I'm too stunned to respond. The question is so unexpected. I've wanted to fire Ida since the beginning but there was no way to tell anyone. Suddenly, I have the chance. Yes, I answer. Get rid of the bitch, but not because of the nose tube. That wasn't her fault. Fire her for slamming me into the rail, for hurting me again and again.

"Are you sure?" Rikki asks.

Yes, I flash. Yes! Yes! Yes!

"I'll do it," she says, leaving to make the call. She's back in a few minutes. "The registry said they would send someone else tonight."

For the first time since this started, I feel powerful. With a shift of my eyes, I've had someone fired. I have an exhilarating sense of control, but Rikki is thoughtful, worried.

"If you could have, would you have fired Ida earlier?" she asks. Yes, I answer.

"You mean you wanted me to get rid of her before today?" Yes.

"Oh, God," she sobs, "the most important question I could ask is how you like the nurses and I never thought of asking." No, I flash, no, no, no! Don't blame yourself, I want to say. You can't think of everything. You're doing great. No one could handle things better.

"Are you happy with Pearl?" Yes and no.

"Do you want me to get rid of her?" she asks, fearfully. No. One fired nurse is enough for now.

"Every day from now on," she vows, "I'm going to ask you if you're happy with your nurses."

The resident is back. He's brought another doctor, an older man with him. I hope this bastard knows what he's doing. "I hear they're having trouble giving you a new nose tube," he says with a charming smile. He asks Rikki to wait outside. Why hadn't anyone suggested that before? It would have saved her much pain.

The new doctor tries the right nostril first. "There's some kind of obstruction," he says.

"Did you ever have a broken nose?" asks Ingrid. No. Jesus, no. It's my deviated septum.

"I'm going to put this in his left nostril," the doctor says.

"Dr. Schick wants it in the right," the resident reminds him.

"I'll explain to Dr. Schick why we couldn't do it."

He slides the tube smoothly up my right nostril but once more it's in my mouth, not my stomach. I'm flashing again. Jesus!

"Something's wrong," Ingrid tells them.

The doctor's hands are very steady, very soft and very clean. He tries three more times and each time he fails.

"We need a thicker tube," he says finally.

"Dr. Schick wanted this gauge," the resident reminds him.

"She can give him the size tube she wants some other

time. We have to start getting liquids into this man. I don't want him dehydrated."

It's finally over. I'm on my side now. White stuff is flowing through the new tube. It's the same size and in the same nostril as the old tube. All that effort and pain for nothing but at least I'm rid of Ida.

Dr. Schick wanted to change tubes to reduce my secretions. I doubt if it would have made a difference. I had just as many secretions before I had a tube in my nose.

It's Pearl's shift now. Before she left, Rikki tuned the radio to a classical music station. A Beethoven symphony is playing. Pearl asks if she can change the station. No, I want to hear this.

"Thanks," she says, switching to the easy listening elevator music she favors, and once again proving she doesn't know her left from her right.

She's at dinner now. Before she left she turned me toward the wall. There's popular Christmas music on her station now. I despise that stuff. It has all the warmth of a Christmas card from an insurance agent. I enjoy sacred Christmas music despite my atheism. Let's put the Christ back into Christmas, I say, at least musically. Auntie Cline would be proud.

"Peace on earth, good will toward men, blah, blah, blah." I sense a movement. There's someone here in the room. It's probably a floor nurse checking on me. A rough hand grabs my shoulder, turns my head. Holy shit, it's Ida!

"Why did you let them fire me?" she demands, her voice an angry hiss. Christ, I'm scared. She can easily kill me. All she has to do is turn off the alarm, disconnect the respirator and walk away.

"I didn't do nothing to you," she says. The fuck you didn't. I start to move my eyes to argue. That's suicidal. Don't let her think you're talking back. Stare, just stare.

"I took good care of you. I bathed you every night. Always saw you were suctioned." As long as she keeps talking she won't do anything dangerous. "I'm a good nurse," she says. "You shouldn't have fired me."

She peers down at me, blinking back tears. She's hurt, really hurt. It doesn't occur to her that she's hurt me many times. "No one's ever fired me," she says. I stare back, unblinking, terrified. I take no pleasure from her pain. Finally, she turns and leaves the room. I won, I guess. I hope she never comes back.

I've come to this hospital for plasmapheresis treatments. They are supposedly more effective if you get them early. In the daily struggle to keep me alive everyone seems to have forgotten that, except for Charlie and me.. I hear Charlie's voice on the tape badgering Rikki to get them to start the treatments. He's away but he hasn't forgotten why I'm here. He's telling Rikki to push Dr. Ramsbotham to get them going. When she finally does he says that they'll start "soon."

It annoys Ingrid that I am constantly asking her to turn me or move my legs. She's lazy and doesn't want to be troubled. She says we should get a mechanical bed that will rock me back and forth. She claims it will be for my comfort. "It will be like being in a hammock," she tells us. Or in a cradle, I think.

The motorized bed idea also appeals to Dr. Schick. She thinks it will help my lungs and circulation. The bed alone costs as much as a luxury hotel room but insurance will pay they tell us reassuringly. Get it!

This is a teaching hospital. On many mornings strange doctors squeeze as many of their students as they can into my tiny room. They use me to lecture on Guillain-Barré. The students look bored. They stare and I stare back. I look for pretty girls but there are not many among these medical students.

The subject for today's class is the long-promised plasmapheresis treatments. "They experimented with it on Guillain-Barré patients in Boston," the doctor tells his students with complete assurance, "and they found the treatments did no good. I don't know why they're bothering with it for him."

His words are chilling. He looks and sounds smarter than Dr. Ramsbotham and he speaks with a tone of absolute certainty. But I can't let him discourage me. Dr. Ramsbotham is the Guillain-Barré expert. Who is this other guy? What does he know? Screw him. Forget what he said.

I can move my hand! It is on my hip under the covers but I'm waving it from side to side. I'm facing the wall but I must be moving the blanket. I'm surprised neither Ingrid nor Rikki have noticed. I'm so happy. Wait until Rikki sees it!

When they turn me it will be obvious to both of them. I flash to be turned. Rikki notices that. They pull the covers back. Ingrid is talking, telling another tale about how she outsmarted a doctor and saved a patient. Now I am uncovered, waving my hand. I can't lift my arm but I can jerk my hand back and forth. Every American boy should be able to do that.

They keep chatting as if nothing special is going on. If they don't see it, maybe it's not happening. Amputees often "feel" missing limbs. Maybe this is the same thing. They couldn't miss seeing my hand move. It seems so real to me but I know it can't be. I'm disappointed.

Rikki slips a picture of us in Paris out of a manila envelope. We're standing in a park with Notre Dame's flying buttresses in the background. I can't bear looking at it. It brings back the memory of that week, of walking down Parisian streets, of romantic dinners and continental breakfasts in our funny little hotel lobby.

"Should I put it here," Rikki asks, holding it up to a spot near the head of my bed. Tears fill my eyes. No, no, no! Take it away. I can't look at it. It makes me too sad.

"I understand how you feel," says Rikki. "I cried too when I first saw the picture. I didn't want to look at it. Then I decided it shows you healthy, standing up—the way you'll be soon again. Please let me put it up, darling."

No, no, no! I don't want to see it. Take it away. "I hope you'll change your mind," she says, sliding the picture into the envelope.

Connie and Ronnie, the plasmapheresis technicians, are here. They know their names sound funny together and that people tend to confuse them. They enjoy that. They're in their mid-twenties and have long been best friends. They went to nursing school together, married their high school boyfriends about the same time and now live in the same New Jersey town. They also quit nursing together to become technicians. It gives them the weekends off to be with their husbands, they say.

One is tall, lanky, and beautifully blonde. The other is shorter, rounder and very cute. They tend to finish each other's sentences. I'm confused about who is who but it doesn't matter. I love them both and trust them completely. They're a set. How could you marry just one?

When they begin the treatments, they explain, they'll put a needle into a vein in one of my arms and draw my blood through a tube to a centrifuge. It'll spin it around to separate and remove the plasma. What's left of the blood is pumped out of the centrifuge, and back into my other arm.

The theory behind all this assumes that there's something wrong with the plasma part of my blood. Removing it will stimulate my body to make new, healthy plasma and I'll regain my strength. How is this different from the old practice of "bleeding" the patient?

They say the treatments are painless. That's good. They examine my arms. Lousy veins, they observe. All their patients have lousy veins, they joke. The needles could leave scars. Christ, I don't want scars on my arms. I don't want to look like a street junkie. They'll return tomorrow morning.

Rikki sits by my bed. "You're going to make a complete recovery," she says. This has become her chant, her litany. Yes, I flash. "You know you'll make a complete recovery?" Yes, I know.

Ingrid sometimes acts as though she and I are very intimate, as if we're former lovers. "You can tell me the truth," she says when we're alone. "Do you really think you'll make a full recovery? Whatever you tell me, I won't tell Rikki."

Why you conniving bitch! Of course you'll tell her. That's why you're asking. You'd love to say, "Bob doesn't think he'll recover. He lies to you so you'll feel better. He's only honest with me."

Actually, you don't give a fuck about me. You just want to cause trouble and come between us. Ingrid, you're pathetic. Yes, I flash, I'm sure I'll make a full recovery. Now go tell Rikki that.

I can refuse the plasmapheresis, the beautiful Dr. Rossi explains. She sounds as if she's reading a prisoner his rights.

"Is there any danger?" Rikki asks.

"None that's known," she says, implying that someday I may have reason to regret this decision. She seems to be straining to sound neutral. I believe that she thinks the treatments are useless.

The decision is mine, she says. I think she wants me to refuse but I can't do that. I have to have the treatments even though I'm losing faith in their doing any good. I must try anything that could make me better. I've come all this way, waited all this time. I have to go through with it.

"The choice is yours," she says, but I have no choice.

"Some of your plasma will be frozen," she tells me. "Years from now researchers may use it to study Guillain-Barré and other diseases."

I start fantasizing -- the year 2015. A young scientist in a spotless modern laboratory peers through a microscope. "Eureka!" he cries. "We cracked the code with the Samuels plasma." Hot dog! Give that man a Nobel Prize.

The new day is tense with anticipation. There's a call on the tape from Charlie. "You can do it Bob!" he chants. "You can do it!" He sounds as if he actually believes the treatments will work. Maybe he's right. If he believes, why shouldn't I? I'll do it for him.

I may get dizzy, even pass out, Connie and Ronnie warn. I'm to signal if I want to stop. But I am determined not to stop no matter what happens. I will go on. It's for Charlie, I decide.

I'm on my back, arms spread Christ-like. The needles are in. The centrifuge hums, spinning at tremendous speed. A clear plastic tube fills with my blood. It is painless. Ronnie and Connie hover over me like angels. They speak to each other in a scientific shorthand. I can't follow it. Am I all right, they ask periodically. Yes, I flash. Yes.

They're taking a relatively small amount of blood this time. On subsequent treatments they'll take more. You have to build up to it. My head spins. "You all right?" one of them asks. Yes, yes! Go!

You can do it, Bob, you can do it!

Oh, Jesus, I need suctioning. I'm choking, drowning, my head's spinning. Now I'm flashing. They see it immediately.

"Should we stop?" the short one asks, thinking I want to quit because I'm dizzy. No, I flash.

"Do you need suctioning?" asks the other. Yes. She suctions lovingly, caringly. I wish they were my nurses. The treatment goes on and on. It's nauseating like an unpleasant ride in an amusement park. Don't stop. This is for Charlie.

It's over. They put big, loose bandages on the crooks of my arms where the needles were. I hope I won't have drug-addict scars.

"Do you feel any different?" Rikki asks. No, tired, just tired. I close my eyes but, of course, I'm not actually closing my eyes. I'm rolling my pupils up in my head. I can't close my eyes.

Go away, please. I want to rest. Maybe I slept a little last night. I'm not sure. The nurse was some young woman who came all the way from Princeton, New Jersey. Her husband is a graduate student there. She was good. I trusted her but she can't be my permanent nurse. She works only occasionally.

Dr. Ramsbotham wakes me. The first time that I'm certain I've been asleep in all this time and he shakes my shoulder!

"Try and move your feet, sir," he asks politely. I try. I always try. He's a fucking madman. He's obsessed with my feet. "Lift an arm, sir." If only I could. Oh, Jesus!

"I didn't expect results, not actually, but one hopes," he explains, red-faced because he guesses I think he's a clown. "Don't despair, sir," he says, patting my hand. "There will be more treatments." It's hard to be angry with him. He is a nice man, a sweet, old English eccentric.

The mechanical bed has finally arrived—the first event to break the monotony in the days since the plasmapheresis. The bed is too large for them to squeeze into this room so they're putting it in one on the sixth floor. Rikki and Ingrid have been going upstairs all day to check on it.

Now Rikki is back. She's actually ridden in the bed and is trying to describe it. "It's like a hammock," she says. "It rocks you back and forth. It keeps you constantly moving. I think you're going to love it."

Ingrid is bubbling with happiness: "You won't want to be turned all the time." What she means is she won't have to turn me all the time.

I'm anxious to try it but there are countless delays. The people leasing it to the hospital want to see that they put me into it the right way but they've wandered off somewhere.

Ingrid's shift is ending. She won't be in tomorrow— she's taking several days off. God knows who they'll send to replace her. Pearl is here now and Rikki has to run. Friends have asked her and Marilyn to dinner. "I hope you love the bed," she says, kissing me as she goes.

Everything is finally ready. I'm on a stretcher. They're pushing me through the halls and onto an elevator. Now they're lifting me into the bed. There seems to be stirrups for my feet and my back is against something that feels like a sling. It's difficult for me to see it.

The manufacturer's representatives are explaining the bed to Pearl. It's fiendishly complicated but even if it were simple I doubt if Pearl could follow what they are saying. There are several other nurses here. Hope they understand.

One of the bed company reps is also a nurse. She calls Pearl Hon. Her male sidekick is a slick sales type. It's late and they're in a rush to leave. There are no doctors around to watch this thing work.

Mr. Sales starts the bed. "Don't be scared," he says, "you can't fall out." Up it goes; the room seems to tilt. It's like seeing the horizon from a banking airplane. I'm not scared, just apprehensive. It sure feels as if I could fall. Down it comes. "See how nice that is." he says. Whee!

The bed is rocking up the other way. Jesus, it's weird. Don't know if I like it or not. Don't judge yet. Wait. Hey, the bed people are gone. They're not staying long enough to see if there are problems. Oh Jesus, the bed's motion has pulled respirator hose off my neck. Beep, beep, beep. Pearl manages to stick it back on.

Two more swings and the fucking hose is unplugged again. Pearl is frantically chasing me with it as I rock slowly past her. I've become a moving target, as if things weren't already tough enough. Come on Pearl catch me! My fingers tingle from lack of oxygen. Bingo, she hits the target with the hose and I inflate. Give that girl a Kewpie doll!

Jesus, now I need suctioning. How is she ever going to see my eyes moving while I'm swinging by her like a slow motion Tarzan? Beep, beep! She's chasing me with the hose again. I'm flashing. She sees I need suctioning. This is insane!

Hurry, Pearl, I can't breathe—I'm drowning. She can't find the goddamn catheters. Everything is in a different place in this room. Now she has a catheter but, Sweet Jesus, she doesn't know how to stop the bed. I'm choking. Hurry, please hurry! The hose is off again. Beep, beep, beep, beep! A nurse is rushing in to help. She's stopping the bed, reattaching the hose. One breath, two breaths, three—now Pearl suctions me. Thank God!

This new nurse is the head nurse for the floor. She's showing Pearl how to start the bed. Off I go into the wild blue yonder, climbing high into the sky. I rock once, twice, and the damn respirator hose pops off. They're stopping the bed to reattach it.

Two more cycles and the fucking hose is off again. The head nurse is thumbing through the bed's manual. "There is nothing here about respirators," she reports.

They launch me again. Two complete swings and I'm detached once more, an astronaut adrift in space without oxygen. The head nurse tries tying the hose to the bed with a pillowcase. Her idea is to have it swing with the bed. That seems to work. Two swings, three, four. Beep, beep, beep. Oh, Jesus, it's off again!

She tries tying it to different parts of the bed, but nothing she does is completely successful. She phones the bed company but no one is there. It's late.

The evening shift is ending. Both Pearl and the head nurse are going off duty. Pearl looks completely frazzled. I feel sorry for her.

We're still having trouble finding someone to work Ida's old midnight to eight shift. Tonight's nurse is a short, plump, pleasant-looking black woman in her fifties. We've never met.

She tries hard to understand all of Pearl's explanations but no one could follow them. It's hard enough taking care of me without having me swinging back and forth.

There's absolutely no chance of me sleeping tonight. The damn tube is coming off all the time and, this new nurse is continually shining a flashlight in my eyes. She's afraid of missing my signals. She's sure trying, but I'm impossible. First I need suctioning, and then I need to be catheterized. The nurse has a friend in a nearby room who helps her. Thank goodness for the friend. Otherwise she would be in tears.

Damn, the terrible sweats are back. Now she has to bathe me. She stops me swinging. The manual says you have to unzip some panels to wash my back. This whole bed is absolutely nutty, designed by Rube Goldberg.

At first it goes well. Then she unzips the part by my backside. I'm slipping out! My bare ass is sticking through the bed, like the stuffing bursting through the casing of a bratwurst, the white German sausage. Christ, this is undignified—obscene. What if I were the Chief Justice of the Supreme Court or Queen Elizabeth? Would they do this to them? What madman invented this bed?

The nurse is crawling under it to wash my ass. With each of these beds they should supply one of those rolling dollies mechanics use to get under a car. Now she's trying to shove my rear end back up into the bed. She's just a little woman. She can't do it. She calls her friend.

This would be funnier if it weren't starting to hurt. They need more help. They get a floor nurse. Now there are three women under me trying to stuff my ass back in place. Someone should take movies.

One of the nurses has her shoes off and is shoving my bare fanny up with her bare feet. It's working! Little by little she's jamming my ass back into the hammock. When it's there, they quickly zip me in.

It's still dark when Rikki arrives. "Couldn't sleep," she explains. "I wanted to know if you like the bed." No!

"Why not?" she asks as the hose pulls off once more. It's been happening all night, the night nurse tells her, adding that she won't take care of me again. "You need a younger woman for this," she declares. Can't blame her. Wish I could quit too.

The bed is a nightmare. My new day nurse, a Trinidadian, can't cope with it either. To keep the respirator hose and me together, it takes her full attention, Rikki's help and constant advice from the floor nurses.

I wish Ingrid were around to struggle with this mess. This bed is her dumb fucking idea. And where is Dr. Schick? She pushed for the bed too. It's Saturday. No chance of her showing up. Doctors don't work Saturdays.

Snap! Jesus, what's that? The cast iron control handle for the bed has broken off. The bed still works but its speed is more difficult to control.

They've called the bed company and it's sending a repairman from Philadelphia. Philadelphia! No one can believe it. Even on a Saturday without traffic that's at best a two-hour drive.

Time for another bath. A floor nurse, who was at yesterday's training sessions, happens to be in the room. She tells them that to wash my back, they have to stop the bed toward the top of a swing. "That way you won't be fighting gravity when you zip him back in," she explains, clearing up the mystery of why they had so much trouble last night.

The repairman from Philadelphia has finally arrived. He replaces the broken handle. They ask him how to keep the respirator hose attached to me. He hasn't a clue. Not his department.

He's been gone ten minutes and up I swing and stop. "I didn't touch anything. Something's stuck," my nurse says. "It's not my fault." She's almost shouting. Jesus, now what?

No one can figure out what's wrong. It's just not moving— it's frozen, paralyzed like me. My left side is up and my right side is down. They can't reach the repairman now. Even when they do, is he going to want to drive back from Philadelphia? I'm getting more uncomfortable. I'm flashing. I want to get out of this bed now.

"Do you want to be suctioned?" asks Rikki. No!

"Has some part of you moved?" No!

"Scratched?" No!

"What do you want?" she cries. "I don't know what you want!"

I want to get out of this fucking bed, I scream to myself. Can't you guess that? I'm sick of it. I've tried it and it doesn't work.

"Do you want the light off?" No! Sometimes lights bother me.

"Do you want to be suctioned?" No! I already said I didn't, Goddamn it!

"Do you want to be moved?" she asks. Yes, that's it!

"Your legs?" No!

"Arms?" No!

"What else can I move?" she asks desperately. Then, suddenly, she knows. "You want to be taken out of this bed?"

Yes! Yes! Yes!

~

It is not a simple matter. They put me in this wacky bed on doctor's orders and they need doctor's orders to get me out. A resident can't order it. It has to be one of my doctors. The floor nurses are phoning both Dr. Ramsbotham and Dr. Schick at home but they get no answer. They'll keep trying.

Rikki stands holding my hand, stroking my face. She has to stand because I'm stuck so high that if she sits she can't see or reach me. "Are you comfortable?" she asks. No!

"Should I do anything about it?" No. So far I can tolerate the pain.

She reads me letters and plays the tape to pass the time. There is a call from my father. He sounds old and depressed. He's grown frail these past few years. When he walks, he uses a colorful Mexican cane. He clowns with it, twirls it like a vaudevillian, but the sad fact is he needs the cane to walk.

We've resolved our father and son conflicts. Old age has brought a new gentleness and sweetness to him. Every parting we have saddens me. His death is no longer inconceivable to me but I want him to live forever. I want us to be old men together. He's my best friend.

He's trying to sound cheerful but his voice betrays him. It tells me my illness has crushed him. He's taken so many blows. How could life, which he's loved so much, do this to him? How could I do this to him? He tells Rikki she's the bravest woman the world has known since Joan of Arc. He doesn't speak to me. He doesn't realize that I'll hear his words.

"Take care of yourself, dear," he tells her. Take care of yourself, Daddy, I want to say. I won't die on you like everyone else. I'm going to be okay. Don't let anything happen to you. We'll see you in February.

Before my eyes can fill with tears, I flash Rikki. "You want them to try the doctors again?" she guesses. Yes!

Neither doctor answers. Rikki knows Dr. Ramsbotham lives in a nearby apartment. She wants to go there and try to find him. Even if he's not home, she thinks that maybe his doorman or a neighbor can tell her where he is. The nurses say they don't have the address, but even if they did they couldn't give it out. She tries the phone book but he's not listed.

I flash repeatedly. I can't tolerate the pain. Rikki runs to the nurses' station. "You must take my husband out of that bed!" But they won't do it. They say they need orders. What happens if my doctors are away for the weekend? Will they let me hang here like a bat until Monday? Rikki clutches my hand. "Don't worry, my darling. I won't leave you."

It seems like hours since the bed broke. My side is stiff with pain. I'm flashing. I won't stop until they get me out of this bed. I'm throwing a tantrum with my eyes. Move me, I scream.

"You have to get my husband out of that bed!" Rikki yells at the nurses. They again patiently explain that they need doctor's orders. "I want to speak to someone in charge!" she yells. She sounds insane, out of control and they seem so reasonable. Rikki is embarrassing me, but that's crazy. I don't want her to stop yelling.

There's a whole crowd of nurses in the room now. One of them says she's in charge of the floor but she can't do anything to help.

"Yes you can. Get him out of that bed!" roars Rikki.

"Mrs. Samuels, we're going to have to ask you to leave."

"You'll have to throw me out," Rikki growls, backing into a corner like a wild animal.

Time out. They're calling a nursing supervisor. The buck needs passing. The supervisor, a stoic, heavy-set woman listens calmly to the whole story.

"You can't leave Mr. Samuels suspended like this." she says finally. "Let's get him down. I'll take the responsibility." Sanity reigns!

Pearl is here. She is delighted the bed is gone. Rikki is ready to go home. She's been in this room more than twelve hours. What would have happened if she hadn't come, if she hadn't yelled, if I had been alone?

Dr. Schick is disappointed that I'm not in the bed. "Will you try it again if I get you an entirely new bed?" she asks sweetly, after hearing that the first one broke.

No, I flash. No! No! No!

"You know I can't force you to change your, mind," she says, "but you should understand that the bed has great therapeutic value. It will help clear up your pneumonia and also help your circulation."

Did anyone tell her that the respirator hose kept coming detached? Did they note it in my chart?

"I'm very surprised at your lack of cooperation," she adds, looking at me like a disappointed schoolteacher.

Dr. Ramsbotham also doesn't understand what is wrong with the bed but he approves of my rebellion. "This is the first time Mr. Samuels is being assertive," he tells Rikki. "That's a good sign."

It turns out I do benefit from the bed because they're letting me stay in this large single room. What luxury! The room has two windows and a bathroom. It even has a phone.

Ingrid loves the phone. Once Rikki leaves for the day, she's on it like a teenager, calling everyone she knows. She holds the receiver near me. "Hear that?" she asks her friends. "That's the sound of the respirator keeping my patient alive." She must believe that this makes her seem like Florence Nightingale.

Now she's telling her roommate about last night's date. "The guy was pitiful," she laughs. "He was begging for it. I told him that I just got my period but even that didn't turn him off. Finally I went down on him just to shut him up."

Does Ingrid forget that I'm here, able to understand everything? Or is she trying to turn me on? Sometimes when we're alone she's very suggestive. "I can't wait until you're well enough to go out in the garden with me. We'll have very deep discussions," she says huskily.

Plasmapheresis time again! It's the second of five planned treatments. Connie and Ronnie have my circulatory system plugged into their machine. God, they're nice. The centrifuge hums. My plasma fills a plastic bag. It looks like urine. My head spins. You can do it, Bob! You can do it!

It's over. Connie and Ronnie are packing up. I'm exhausted. So far the treatments are useless but I'll keep having them. I've got to try anything. Plasmapheresis attracts flies to my room. Flies in December! Jesus, I'm tired.

Two nurses are visiting me. "You're going to get better," one of them is saying. "Don't let anyone tell you you ain't, you understand?" she asks, shaking my hand to keep me awake. Yes, I answer. She has a Brooklyn accent, like my father's. I'm so sleepy. "I've taken care of lots of folks like you. They've all gotten better," she continues. I'm drifting off.

Pearl still struggles with the respirator. She leaves me off it too long. Fortunately, most of the time she also forgets to silence the warning beep. It brings someone running to see what's wrong at least once a shift.

I'm off the machine so often that I sometimes fear that I may have suffered brain damage from lack of oxygen. I test myself. I'm able to recall names of people at Texaco whom I barely know, every curve and landmark on seldom used highways and the interiors of houses I visited years ago. I guess I'm still okay.

Water from condensation collects in the respirator hoses. Mostly it settles in the main one, running from my neck to the machine. The nurse usually empties it when she suctions me. Shorter hoses connect other parts of the machine. Those are cleared by respiratory technicians who visit my room to service the machine at least three times every 24 hours.

There's an annoying gurgling in one of the hoses tonight and it's bothering Pearl. She's not sure where the sound is coming from. She detaches the hose from my neck. Beep, beep, beep... She shakes it but only a few drops come out. Beep, beep, beep... Now she's tearing the shorter hoses off the machine. Holy shit, Pearl, you don't know what you're doing! Beep, beep, beep... I can't breathe! She'll never get everything back together again.

Beep, beep, beep... She's staring in dumb amazement at the fucking machine, as if she's never seen it before. I'm tingling from lack of oxygen. My vision is dimming. It's like someone has turned down the lights. Beep, beep, beep...

I'm losing consciousness. I'm going to die. Jesus, I'm amazingly calm about it. Hope Rikki gets a good lawyer and sues the asses off these bastards. Now a black void, nothingness, death.

"Mr. Samuels! Wake up, Mr. Samuels!" Some son-of-a-bitch is shouting, shaking my shoulder with an iron grip. It's a tall, lanky guy in surgeon's clothes. He needs a shave. When he sees I'm awake, he releases me. "He'll be okay now," he says, leaving abruptly. Case closed. Next crisis! My shoulder aches from his grip.

The group of curious nurses drifts away from my room. One of them must have come to investigate the beep and found me unconscious and called for help. If Pearl were slightly more competent she would have turned off the beep and I'd have stayed dead. Pearl looks bewildered. I don't think she comprehends what she did, even now.

Dr. Ramsbotham is here with a woman in a party dress. "Is Mr. Samuels all right?" he asks. I'm fine, Pearl tells him. "I was upstairs at the faculty Christmas party when I heard there was an arrest," he tells us. "Was there trouble with the respirator?"

"Yes," says Pearl.

"You did the right thing," he assures her. "It wasn't your fault." What the fuck does he mean! Whose fault does he think it was? Does he think the machine came apart on its own? Does he think I was trying to commit suicide?

"This is Mrs. Ramsbotham," he tells us, remembering his manners. "She was at the party with me." Mrs. Ramsbotham, a pale, shy-looking woman smiles hesitantly. "Well good night, sir," he tells me. "I'll let you rest now."

"You did the right thing," he again tells Pearl, patting her arm. Dr. Ramsbotham, you're a bumbling asshole! If you're the best doctor in New York for Guillain-Barré, God help the rest.

Pearl is on her meal break. A floor nurse is in the room. "You want to get rid of Pearl, don't you?" she asks. Yes, I flash. "Don't worry," she says.

"Something happened last night," Ingrid tells Rikki the next morning.

"What do you mean?"

"There was an emergency of some kind. It's hard to understand from the chart because they don't want us to know but I can read between the lines."

"Is it true? Did something happen?" Rikki asks me. Yes. She questions me no more. She'd rather not know and I don't blame her.

Ingrid is back from lunch, breathless with excitement. "Pearl's been taken off the case!" she tells us. "I ran into her at the registry and she was very upset. She said what happened wasn't her fault. I told her I didn't know what happened but I couldn't get her to explain."

"Was what happened Pearl's fault?" Rikki asks me.

Yes! Yes! Yes!

I'm moving my hand again but nobody sees it. It has to be my imagination. They're not all blind. When will I really move it? When will I start getting better? When will I go home? I miss it so.

Because we're paying for my phone and not using it, Rikki has had them remove it. Now, instead of making calls after Rikki leaves, Ingrid turns on the National Public Radio show *All Things Considered*. Today, noting it is the shortest day of the year, they play a tape from a woman in rural Alaska. She's recorded herself running up a hill behind a dog sled, trying to get to catch a glimpse of the low winter sun as it peeks over the horizon. She's describing what she sees and feels in the arctic half-light. I hear the yelp of the dogs, the crunch of the snow and her breath, which comes in great gulps. She's straining to keep up with her dogs in the clear, cold air.

The contrast to my circumstances couldn't be greater. I'm a flaccid heap, lying in an overheated room in one of the world's largest cities. If it wasn't for machines and other people, I couldn't survive. I want to run up a snowy hill with my dog. Maybe before winter is done I will.

Rikki tells me that people are starting to think that I may be in even worse condition than I am because she's kept them away. I don't want them thinking that. I hadn't wanted them to see me in that small, awful room. It made me look like a charity case.

"Will you see anyone from Texaco?" Rikki asks. No, I fear that they wouldn't believe that I can bounce back quickly from this. I don't want them to take my job away.

Max Riggsbee, the Nyack High School guidance counselor, and his friend Phyllis Mathis, a teacher, are the first of the new visitors. Rikki has told them what to expect but it's not hard for me to see that my respirator and tubes make them nervous. Max can't stop talking; Phyllis says very little. Jesus, am I that bad?

There's something sharp stabbing into my ribs but as long as they're here I'll ignore it. I don't want to upset them. I want to be polite. Max is yakking about a trip to St. Louis he's planning for some conference.

I wish they'd leave now so I could ask to get off this thing. Jesus, are they ever going to go? What the fuck am I lying on, a railroad spike? I can't bear the pain any longer. I'm flashing. Rikki help me!

Do I want to be suctioned, she asks, starting through the list, demonstrating to them how efficiently we communicate. No. Legs moved? No. Arms? No. Is the pillow okay? Yes. Lights? Yes. Is something wrong below my waist? No. Above my waist? Yes. I was just turned so she doesn't ask about that.

More questions. Her frustration is growing. Max and Phyllis are making worried suggestions but they can't begin to guess what's wrong. Rikki is calling Ingrid from the nurses' lounge.

Get me off this fucking spike! It's pushing through my ribs! More questions. "Are you lying on something?" Ingrid finally guesses. Yes! Yes! Yes!

They all watch in horror as Ingrid rolls me off my side. "Here's the problem," she says brightly. She's so proud to be the one clever enough to figure it out. It turns out that I've been lying on a disposable syringe that she misplaced after my last heparin shot. She doesn't say she's sorry. She doesn't have the sense to be embarrassed.

After Rikki has gone, Jon Feller, a photographer friend from Nyack, unexpectedly drops in. He's in his early fifties with silvery hair and boyish Ivy League good looks. He's been divorced for years. Women are attracted to him. Ingrid is no exception. She quickly turns the radio off.

As they discuss me, they flirt. Soon I'm forgotten. They're asking each other personal questions. Their looks grow deeper, fraught with meaning. They're like the couple in the "Tom Jones," movie, lustily eyeing each other while devouring a roast chicken. Now I know how that chicken felt.

"I'll be waiting when your shift ends," he tells her.

"Yes," she sighs. They've shown remarkable self-restraint.

The next afternoon Ingrid casually announces, "I'm moving to Nyack to live with Jon." Lots of luck, Jon!

Because Ingrid doesn't have time for both Jon and me, two days later, I get a new day nurse, Clare Ann Byrne. She showed up unannounced this morning and reminded me that she visited me after a plasmapheresis treatment. Do I remember? Yes, she was the one with a Brooklyn accent like my father's. Thank you, Jon!

Clare Ann has wanted to be my nurse ever since she overheard two doctors discussing my case on an elevator. She sought out Ingrid then and told her that if she wanted to quit, she would be interested in taking over. Ingrid had told her that she would stick with me until I recovered.

Clare Ann had almost forgotten about me. Then, last night, Ingrid phoned unexpectedly to ask if she still wanted the job. Ingrid said commuting from Nyack for the day shift was too difficult. Clare Ann said yes. Ingrid will fill the opening on the evening shift. It all seems too good to be true.

Clare Ann Byrne is an extraordinarily competent nurse. She quickly takes charge. She's going to contact someone she knows to work the night shift. She's also logically and meticulously reorganizing my room. What a change from Ingrid! Finally, says Rikki, we have someone looking after us and we don't have to worry each day about finding nurses.

Like all private duty nurses, Clare Ann is a freelancer. Most take the first case that comes their way but she tries to specialize in nursing acutely ill neurological patients, particularly Guillain-Barré victims. She prefers them because they always recover. Damn right! How fortunate she found me. Why didn't the hospital or my doctors find her for me?

Clare Ann has rules. Rule one is no one calls her Clare. The name is Clare Ann. She's also very rigid about other people's names. Rikki is Mrs. Samuels. I'm Robert, not Bob.

She is pale and petite and seems to be in her late thirties. Her eyes are her best feature. They are deep set and bright green. I've never been able to believe that green eyes are real. Her naturally blonde hair is just long enough to cover her ears. Despite all these attractive features she just misses being pretty. Her single failing is a long upper lip.

"You know," she says, "I ain't gonna turn you every time you ask. I don't know what you're used to but the rule is you're supposed to be turned once every two hours."

Every two hours! Who made that rule? I can't survive for two hours without being turned! "Did you know that's what they do here in intensive care, Robert?" No, I flash.

"Well, that's the rule up there. They don't have time to baby the patients," she lectures. I can't wait two hours for you to turn me. I just can't.

"Because you're used to being turned whenever you want," she continues, "I ain't gonna make you wait two hours now. To start, I'll turn you every hour." Thank God!

She turns me. Hot damn, sweet relief. "If you need anything," she tells Rikki, after calling her back into the room, "I'll be in the nurses' lounge."

Rikki is looking everything over. "See the way she's organized it all," she marvels. "She's going to make such a difference."

Jesus, how long does an hour last? I must never have waited that long to be turned. My knees are bent. They're cramped. I flash Rikki. She starts through the list. I stop her when she asks about my legs. "Should I do the exercises?" No, don't hurt your back by pumping my legs. "Should I change their position?" Yes!

That's better. Now I'll make it. Christ, now I need suctioning. Rikki is running to get Clare Ann. She's here in a flash, ordering Mrs. Samuels to wait outside the room. She suctions me perfectly.

"Since I'm here, Robert, I'll turn you even though the hour ain't yet up." She's letting me know that I'm not getting away with anything. I don't care as long as she moves me. "You had to have your wife change your legs," she says sardonically as she pulls back the sheets. She acts as if having Rikki do that is some terrible weakness. As she lectures me, I stare at the line of reindeer marching across her blue ski sweater.

When Dr. Schick stops by on her daily rounds, she greets Clare Ann like an old friend. They've shared many patients, she tells me jovially, adding that Clare Ann is the hospital's best nurse. Why didn't you tell us about her? Why did you keep her a secret? Why did you risk my life with all those fools?

Even Dr. Ramsbotham knows about Clare Ann. He also calls her the best. Didn't he want the best for his patient? He's asking me to move my feet. Clare Ann seems embarrassed for him. She is staring at the ceiling.

Ingrid is late. Day shift, evening shift, it doesn't matter, she's always late. Clare Ann has the room ready for her— everything in its place. She's even coiled the suctioning tube. Rikki has gone home. I want to be turned but I don't dare ask since it hasn't been an hour since the last time. I know Ingrid will turn me. She has no rules. Slobs have their good points.

I see Ingrid's handsome face. I want to signal her to turn me now but I'm afraid if I do Clare Ann will tell her about the every hour rule. They leave the room to talk about me. Come on! I want you to turn me!

Ingrid is finally in the room by herself. I'm flashing like crazy. Let's go! Turn me now! I'm like a dog jumping in circles for attention. "Clare Ann told me to only turn you once an hour," Ingrid tells me. Fuck Clare Ann, her rules and the horse she rode in on! You're here now! You're in charge! Turn me!

"Do you think it's been an hour since you were turned the last time?" I lie. Yes! Yes! Yes!

"Oh, well, ok," Ingrid sighs, turning me. She knows nothing about discipline, thank God!

Welcome back Ingrid! She puts nothing away. Within a few hours my room is in turmoil. She and Clare Ann are the "Odd Couple," straight sit-com. More fun for the bored patient but Ingrid is not happy. Without Rikki or anyone else to impress, there is no point to this job. She wanders off, leaving me alone for frighteningly long stretches.

It's midnight and that means new nurse time! It usually fills me with dread but Clare Ann has pre-approved this one so I'm reasonably confident she won't be a lunatic. I hear her voice now. Hey, all right, she's pretty and classy looking. Shiny, expensively cut dark brown hair frames her open, honest face. She has lots of big teeth and a nice wide smile. Her uniform is more stylish than the usual. It has a pleated front covering big, comfortable looking boobs. Her name is Laura DuBois.

When Laura is nervous, her nose wiggles, making her look like a worried rabbit. I don't blame her for being nervous. There is so much to do in this new job. She calls me Robert, a la Clare Ann. I'm flashing. I want her to turn me. I want to see if she's going to give me any nonsense about waiting an hour. No, she turns me.

My bed is a mess. Ingrid didn't even bother to change my sheets. Laura doesn't complain. She finds fresh linen and does it. She's okay, this Laura. As soon as she's made the bed I go into the terrible sweats. That puts Laura's nose in spasms. God, she's frantic, bathing me, changing the bed again. No rest for Laura! She starts cranking up the back of the bed to feed me. They raise it a little every time I'm fed but not this much. Stop! You're going too far. I'm flashing, in pain. Can't stand having you bend my body this much. Put me down! Lower the back of the bed, you bitch!

"The bed has to be elevated," she explains, guessing why I'm upset. "If you vomited and the bed was level the vomit could get in your lungs. It could be fatal."

No! No! I flash. I understand, but you don't have to go this high. No one else does. Please put me down, please.

"I'm not going to lower the bed, until I finish feeding you," she says stubbornly. I flash but she ignores me. She pours a can of white stuff into the plastic bag at the other end of my tube. It flows like molasses. I'm growing cross-eyed watching it ooze down. Finally, it's done. I'm flashing again. Lower the bed, damn it! Lower the bed! "A half-hour more," she declares, her nose vibrating. "You need that long to digest your food."

I'm insane with rage. Are you out of your fucking mind? There's nothing in that crap to digest. If you can't chew it, smell it, or taste it, how the hell can you digest it? Put me down! Put me down! Put me down! Put me down!

"You'll have to wait," she says firmly. The half-hour creeps by. I'm going to fire your ass, Laura. I don't have to take this!

Before the first light of dawn Rikki is here to meet Laura. "What do you think?" she asks me as soon as we're alone. I shift my eyes yes, no, yes, no. "You don't know yet?" she guesses. Yes, that's right. Hours have passed. My temper has cooled. Except for the feeding, she was fine. Maybe tonight she won't put the back of the bed up so high.

"I'll ask you again tomorrow." Rikki promises.

Clare Ann sure has a lot of rules. This is a hospital, she reminds us. Mrs. Samuels must leave the room each time I'm turned, suctioned, or have chest p.t. Mrs. Samuels must not sit on the side of the bed or move the patient in any way. And, of course, Clare Ann will not turn Robert more than once an hour.

She isn't all negatives. She says we should have the TV connected so I won't feel so isolated. I haven't wanted it because I know I won't see the screen clearly without my glasses. And how will I be able to tell anyone what I want to watch. Television is bad enough when you can choose your own programs.

"Do you want me to have it turned on?" Rikki asks after talking to Clare Ann. No, I flash.

When Rikki tells her how I feel, Clare Ann looks exasperated. She doesn't believe in asking patients about anything. "Robert shouldn't be cut off from the world," she argues. She has a good point. I don't want Rikki fighting with her about this so I change my mind. I'll try television.

There is a call on the answering service tape from my parents. They're again offering to come to New York. "I called them back," Rikki says, "and told them there would be nothing for them to do here. They couldn't help. You still don't want them, do you?" she asks.

No, I flash. They have lived in Mexico so long that they probably don't even own winter clothes anymore. My father is so frail that I fear a bitterly cold day could kill him. They did come to New York when my sister had her biopsy but it was summertime and my father was stronger. Both Joan and I needed him.

Joan's illness, like mine, came on with a terrible swiftness. She was in fine health until a neighbor found her in convulsions on the floor of her apartment. At Roosevelt Hospital, where she was rushed by ambulance, they thought it might be epilepsy but, after several days of tests, a cat scan revealed a tumor on the left side of her brain. A biopsy was scheduled.

Because she'd never married, Joan and I were unusually close. She treated me like a big brother even though I was more than four years younger. Now she was scared and wanted me to tell her what to do about almost everything. I didn't have the answers. I wanted my father.

When he arrived, I told him all my fears and asked what he thought we should tell Joan if the growth was cancerous. She wasn't a strong or brave person. How could she live with such awful news?

"We can't tell Joan," he said flatly.

"What do you mean we can't tell her? She'll want to know. You don't keep things like that from people these days."

"Joan won't want to know," he predicted.

Joan's doctor suggested we wait at her apartment, which was not far from the hospital. He promised to phone us with the results of the operation. This happened on the day Richard Nixon was leaving the White House for the last time. Rikki and my parents and I joyously watched the television coverage while filled with dread about Joan.

The President of the United States was taking his final ride on Air Force One when the phone rang. Rikki turned down the TV sound as I answered. It was Joan, not her doctor. She was back in her room, wanting to know all about Nixon. She was feeling fine and didn't seem the least concerned about the results of the biopsy. We marveled at her spirit.

That afternoon at the hospital, her neurosurgeon, a sensitive former psychiatrist, gave me the stunningly tragic news. "She has a tumor called an astrocytoma," he said. "We could have operated and gotten most of it and maybe prolonged her life for a while but it would have left her unable to speak. I don't think she'd be happy living that way."

"Isn't there anything you can do?" I asked calmly. I was finding the conversation unreal.

"Yes," he said, "there is. We'll treat her with radiation. That will shrink the tumor but only temporarily. Eventually it will start growing again."

"How long does she have?"

"A year, maybe longer."

"Oh, Jesus."

"It's terrible."

"Will she be in much pain?"

"She shouldn't have any pain. Once the radiation treatments are finished, she'll even be able to return to work and, for a while, resume her normal life."

"My father doesn't think we should tell her the truth," I blurted, expecting him to say my father was ridiculously old-fashioned.

"I think your father is right."

"You do?"

"Yes."

"Well, what do we tell her? I don't think we should lie."

"We don't have to lie."

"What do I say if she asks what's going to happen?"

"Tell her that we have to wait and see. That's all you have to say."

"What if she asks directly, 'Do I have cancer? Am I going to die?'"

"Then you'll have to tell her but let her ask before you do."

Of course, she'll ask, I thought. She'll want to know. How can she not wonder why she's having radiation treatments? She'll ask. I know she will.

She never did. A few times during that year she would cry and tell me she didn't know what was going to happen. I'd hug her and tell her we'd have to wait and see. Even after the second bout of radiation, and the loss of her hair, she didn't press for details. My father had been right. She didn't want to know.

I'm so different.

I'm a realist, a journalist. I want them to tell me everything. Rikki knows that. She tells me the truth.

Fuck you Laura, I howl silently in pain and indignation. You've put the back of the bed even higher than last night. This time you've had it. I can hardly wait to tell Rikki to fire you.

"Was Laura okay last night?" Rikki asks. No, I flash angrily.

"Do you want me to get rid of her?"

Yes, yes! Kick her ass out!

"You don't want to have Laura anymore?" she asks, making sure she has it right.

Yes.

"You know we'll have trouble getting a nurse to replace her?"

Yes, but I don't care. I'll take my chances.

"The registry is trying to find someone else for tonight," she tells me later. "They were surprised things didn't work out with Laura DuBois."

Let them be surprised. "Oh, I almost forgot to tell you," Rikki continues, breaking into a smile, "Charlie called last night. He's driving home this afternoon for the start of his Christmas vacation."

Late afternoon and there's still no Charlie. They've connected the television but we've barely had it on. Rikki has been getting up to look out the window. She hopes to see Charlie parking the car or walking down the street. All I ever see from my bed is some sky. Today, it's dismal and grey.

Rikki is dozing in a chair. Suddenly, Charlie is in the doorway. Rikki is up embracing him. It's dark outside but he fills my room with sunshine, taking it over with his youth and health.

"How you feeling, Bob?" he asks in a big loud voice. "Okay?" Yes.

Clare Ann rushes from the nurses' lounge to see what the noise is about. She does nothing to stop Charlie when he grabs one of my legs and starts pumping it. She must like him like everyone else.

"Hey, your new room even has TV," he says, picking up the remote control and giving it a try. Rikki is leaving for home to make dinner for him.

"I visited a psychiatrist at college to talk about you," he tells me when we're alone. I'm shocked. I never imagined he'd need a psychiatrist. Jesus, all the problems I've caused. Oh, my son, I'm so sorry.

"You know what the psychiatrist told me?" he asks brightening, not sensing my mood. No, I flash. "She told me it was perfectly understandable that I was depressed. She pointed out I really do have problems. My whole life fell apart. She made me feel a lot better."

Yes, yes, I flash, trying to tell him I agree, that I'm applauding the doctor for her good sense.

It shouldn't surprise me that he went to a psychiatrist. Who else do nonreligious people like us have to turn to for solace? Shrinks ease us past life's unknowables—shamans for moderns.

"When I first got back to school," he continues, "it was hard to study, but I'm getting things back under control." Now he's telling me of his plans for next semester. The conversation seems natural even though I can't speak.

Ingrid's here bustling around, trying to impress Charlie, whom she is meeting for the first time. The way she's eyeing him, I'm sure that she'd be after him if she weren't with Jon. Charlie isn't ready for someone like her.

It's late, Charlie's been gone a long time and I'm apprehensive. Ingrid's shift is almost over and I don't know who will relieve her. I'm having second thoughts about firing Laura but I can't turn back now.

The new nurse is a young black woman who doesn't talk to me, seemingly doesn't understand that I can communicate. She handles me indifferently but not, thank God, brutally. I don't like her; don't trust her. She's very cold.

Oh my God! I can't win. I fired Laura for putting the head of the bed up too high, but this one is feeding me without raising it at all. What's wrong with you, you dumb bitch? If I throw up, I'll drown in my own vomit. Your carelessness can kill me. Put the back of the fucking bed up! I don't want to die! I shift my eyes crazily but she notices nothing.

Don't think about it. Fear can make you sick to your stomach. Calm down. The more time that passes, the safer you are. I wait, trying to think of other things. Nothing happens. The danger must be over.

Suddenly there's a group of people here. My nurse and her friends are standing around my bed, talking loudly about me, saying how sick I look. I feel powerless, like a tiny baby lying on the floor of a playpen. They're complaining about never getting lucrative, long-term cases like mine. They say the registry is prejudiced against blacks. I think they're wrong. The registry sends us anyone who can breathe, regardless of race or competency.

Something new—my nurse is catheterizing me while her friends watch. The whole group is laughing and talking loudly, as if it's the middle of the day, not the middle of the night. They're leaving for the cafeteria. There's a yank on my penis. My catheter has slipped out. No one is here to notice.

Much time has passed and no one has been in checking on me. I don't think my nurse told the floor nurses she was leaving. I want to be turned. I want to be taken care of. Why can't I find a good nurse?

Charlie and Rikki are home, asleep, safe. Home seems so far away. Is it possible I'll ever be home again? My eyes fill with tears. I want this nightmare to end.

My nurse is back. She finds the catheter and the half-filled bag of urine on the floor and throws them in the garbage. I don't even want to imagine what's in hospital garbage.

She should catheterize me again. My bladder hasn't emptied. That could cause me to get a bad infection. I shouldn't have all these worries.

"How was the nurse?" Rikki asks in the morning. I swing my eyes left and right, saying so-so. I can't tell her to fire the nurse every morning.

Clare Ann is irate because we let Laura go because she raised the bed too high. "How do you know how high the back of the bed should be?" Clare Ann asks "Are you a nurse?" I don't respond. I know I can't win. "Tell me, are you a nurse?" she repeats, boring in like Mr. District Attorney. No, I flash trying to shut her up. I'm staring at the reindeer on her stupid sweater. Why do you wear the same idiotic sweater every day? I want to ask.

She's also angry at Rikki for listening to me and not consulting with her about the decision. I wish we had. The new nurse is dangerously bad.

Charlie is telling me how sad his friends are over what's happened. Nice kids, his friends. I had great friends at his age too, but these kids seem to care more about each other than we did. They also seem less obsessed with sex. They actually have friends of the opposite gender. His gang seems like a new race, all lean and muscular. Frisbee is their game, not football.

Charlie pumps my legs. I love the movement, the stretching. Can't get enough. He plays the tape of calls. For the moment I'm at peace. Last night's terrors seem far away. "Are you glad you left Nyack?" he asks.

Yes. If I hadn't made the move, I'd have spent the rest of my life wondering if plasmapheresis would have worked.

"The doctors here are better, aren't they?" he asks. Yes, I flash, hiding my doubts.

"And the nurses are better too, right?" I give him my yes-no answer. I don't want him to know how bad things are.

My birthday is the day after tomorrow, Christmas. To celebrate it, Clare Ann plans to dress me in a red hospital gown. She wants Charlie to take a gown home and dye it. He says he'll ask Rikki to help him. "No, don't tell your mother. I want it to be a surprise. You just put red dye in the washing machine," she explains.

Don't do it Charlie. Don't let her dress me like a clown.

"Hide the gown on your way out," she cautions him as he leaves. "We don't want the security guards to see it." I hope they catch him and take it away.

"That nurse you had last night isn't coming," Ingrid tells me when she starts her shift. "They're sending Arthur instead." It was just a week or so ago that Ingrid was telling us that almost all male nurses are gay.

"They're always coming on to their patients," she claimed. That's all I need, some guy touching me. I want to ask her if what she told us is true. I don't want him if there is any chance I'll be molested. What if he rapes me? It would be like screwing a corpse. But there are guys who screw corpses.

Ingrid must be lying about male nurses. It must be just another of her made-up medical horror stories. She told one recently about a dead patient in Baltimore. According to her, one shift put him on a respirator and left him for the next shift so they wouldn't have to do the paper work. I didn't believe that and I don't believe what she said about male nurses. Still, I can't help worrying.

Ingrid's shift is flying by. Before I know it she's introducing me to Arthur, a small man with black curly hair. I try to relax. I have never been homophobic. Arthur doesn't act particularly effeminate. Seems like a bright guy. Talks a lot—too much. Keeps talking about how good a nurse he is. Suddenly he's crossed the line of credibility. He's a con artist. Tells me how he was in charge of an intensive care unit, more an executive than a nurse. I don't believe him and I don't like him.

He assumes he's going to be my permanent night nurse. Says what a great team he and Clare Ann will make, implying I'll have the Ruth and Gehrig of nursing. Wonder where Ingrid fits in this all-star lineup. I flash to be turned.

"Just hold on," he says. "I want to read your chart. Once I read it I'll have it cold." No one could read my chart and have it cold. It's the size of a novel. Still I wait. Have no other choice. I hear pages slowly turn. I'm shifting my eyes rapidly to get his attention but he's still reading the damn chart. Finally, he puts it down. I'm so cramped. Please turn me.

"Okay, I'll turn you," he says. Now I worry about him molesting me. Will his hands slip? Will he touch me in a sexual way? He turns me. His hands are completely impersonal. "I'm checking my watch," he says. "I'll turn you again in two hours."

No, no, I flash.

"Yes, yes," he mimics, sounding effeminate for the first time. "The chart says you're restless and ask to be turned frequently. I'm going to teach you discipline."

No, no discipline! This isn't the Marines. You're my nurse. You're supposed to help me when I need help. He ignores my flashing. Bide your time, I tell myself, something will happen.

Something does happen. My secretions are to the point where he has to suction me. He's up now, he shouldn't mind turning me. I flash, begging to be turned. "You have an hour and ten minutes more," he says smugly.

Mental telepathy doesn't work. I've tried to use it to get attention and no one ever responds. If mental telepathy worked, this bastard would know my suffering and turn me. If it worked, a floor nurse would come in and see me flashing.

Arthur must be sitting down. I can't see him. He could be sleeping. I hate you, you fucking faggot. I will die; I wish I could die!

At last he stirs. I'm flashing like mad—a dog wagging his tail, overjoyed that the master is up. "Two hours are over," he says. "You want to be turned?" Yes, yes, yes! I'm twirling in circles, pissing on the floor with joy.

He hesitates. "I think you need a bath and a linen change." My tail slows. I don't care what you do, just move me, get me off this side. He fills a basin for my bath. He's washing me but he still hasn't turned me. Forget the bath. Turn me now!

Oh, ah, he's turning me. Tears of relief. He's washing my other side. Why must I wait two hours for this? Why? Why?

"Forgot to get linen," he says. "I'll be back in a minute." To hold me on my side, he drapes my arms over the guardrail. At first I think it's a very neat trick, but now it feels like my arms are being pulled from their sockets.

Where did the son-of-a-bitch go? How could he leave me hanging like this? I want to fire him. I want to get rid of all these nurses. I can't stand any of them. Maybe it's my fault, something wrong with me.

Where are you, you fag? Are you having an assignation in the linen closet? The blood has stopped circulating in my arms. My arms throb. It's screamingly painful.

Is someone in the room now? I can't see the door. Arthur, where are you? Help me! I AM A HUMAN BEING, YOU COCKSUCKING BASTARD!

"Had to go to another floor for linens," he explains offhandedly, unhooking my arms. Blood surges through them. I'm burning with hatred and self-pity. My life is reduced to waiting to be rolled over in bed. All I think about is the next turn. Two hours is forever. I am not really like a dog —a dog has more freedom. I wonder if dogs get Guillain-Barré. I love Ruffy but I wish he had this instead of me. No respirators for dogs. Curtains for poor old Ruff.

Where's Arthur? I'm not even sure if he's in the room. Maybe he's meeting his lover back in the linen closet. Rikki's here! Can't believe it. No mental telepathy. Wasn't even thinking of her. I'm flashing a hello. She kisses me. I smell the outdoors, New York, the world.

"Wake up," she's telling Arthur. "Wake up!" she shouts.

"Uh," he says groggily. "Who are you?"

"I'm Rikki, Bob's wife. Who are you?"

"Oh, ah, I'm Arthur. The registry sent me." He's shrinking before my eyes. He's no longer a tyrant teaching me discipline. He's just a frightened little man.

"You were sound asleep."

"I didn't get any rest yesterday," he whines. "I didn't know I'd be working. I didn't think I'd be called."

I'm flashing. "You want to be turned?" Rikki asks. Yes, yes. "Bob wants to be turned," she tells Arthur. He doesn't argue.

"I'm getting rid of him," Rikki says after he leaves. She's so furious that she doesn't even bother to ask my opinion.

"He's one of the best nurses here," says Clare Ann.

"I don't care. He was dead asleep when I got here. If Bob had needed anything, if there had been an emergency, he wouldn't have known. I had to yell to wake him. That's unforgivable."

"He's hard of hearing," Clare Ann explains.

"That's all the more reason for him to stay awake. Am I right?" she asks me. Yes, I flash.

Now we're in real trouble. The registry hasn't found anyone to replace Arthur. It's Christmas Eve so no one wants to work tonight. If she could get Laura to come back, asks Clare Ann, would I accept her? Yes, I flash. If you want me to, I'll kiss her feet. Clare Ann makes the call. Laura will work tonight!

Now we owe Clare Ann and she's going to collect. From now on, she announces, she doesn't want Rikki here before ten am. We're too busy for visitors before then, she says. She's concerned that Rikki is exhausting herself by visiting every day, she claims. She's told me she thinks it would be better for me, better for my character, to spend more time alone. I want a nurse, not a missionary! A character defect didn't put me in this bed.

Rikki and Charlie had planned to visit me first thing Christmas morning. They were then going to pick up my Aunt Frances at her apartment on West 86th Street and bring her to our house for Christmas dinner with Rikki's parents, just as we planned before I got sick.

Can't the new early visiting rules begin after Christmas, Rikki asks. She doesn't want Frances, who is in her eighties and frail, waiting in the car while she and Charlie come up separately to visit me. Clare Ann says no. The new visiting hours begin tomorrow, despite Frances, despite my birthday, despite Christmas. No exceptions!

Rikki could easily win this argument. She has Dr. Ramsbotham's permission to visit anytime, night or day. She holds back, afraid of angering Clare Ann. We don't want her to quit. It would be impossible to replace her and she knows we know that.

It's good to have Laura back. She says nothing about our firing her. I had forgotten the intensity of the pain she'd caused until she cranked up the back of the bed to feed me. I'm trying not to protest but, as Arthur pointed out, I have no discipline. I feel as though she's bending me in half. I don't understand why sitting up is so difficult. I angrily shift my eyes and Laura nervously twitches her nose. I lose again. The bed stays up.

If the bed is the only problem with Laura, I'll suffer with it. In every other way she's fine, even likable. She has a kindness I've found rare in nurses.

My forty-fifth Christmas Day and I'm alone. Clare Ann is out of the room. *Like Scrooge, I'm visited by ghosts of Christmases past. I'm drifting, dreaming of the pony I always wanted. Now I'm five years-old, put to bed after a long day. "Don't touch my fire truck!" I call to my father when I hear its bell tinkle. I'm 10, accidentally slicing open my thumb with a shiny, new Boy Scout knife. There's bright red blood on the new blade's shiny chrome.*

I'm 11 and a blizzard strands my grandmother (my mother's mother) at our suburban house. There's candlelight because the storm has knocked out the power. We crowd around the fireplace and my grandmother tells us wonderful stories about coming from Russia to America as a child. I'm twenty-one, in the Air Force in Alaska. KP for Christmas...

A sudden, terrifying roar startles me. It's some very loud do-gooder dressed as Santa Claus Ho! Ho! Hoing! to cheer up the patients. My heart doesn't resume its normal rhythm until Charlie arrives. "You brought the gown?" Clare Ann asks. He hands it to her. It's a sad, washed out red.

"See how great your father looks," she says, calling Charlie back into the room after she has it on me. He smiles appreciatively but as soon as she leaves he asks if I like it. No, I don't. He's not surprised.

"Rikki said you'd hate it but she said we should to go along with Clare Ann. Do you agree?" Yes.

He unwraps his present to me. It's a copy of "Tapestry," the great Carole King album. We'd worn out the old one and I'd always meant to replace it. He remembered. "You like your present?" Yes, it's a great present. "You'll be home soon listening to it." Yes. He must go now and sit in the car with Frances.

I stare at the door until I see Rikki. Colorfully wrapped presents fill her arms "Merry Christmas, darling! Happy birthday, my love!" I feel the dampness of her tears as she kisses me. "I know you hate wearing that damn thing," she says, fingering my red gown. Yes, yes, yes, you understand.

"Through all of this you haven't changed a bit have you darling?" she asks, embracing me with a sob. "Inside there is still the Bob I know and love?" Yes, yes, yes. I'm still here, still me.

She opens presents ordered long before any of this happened. There's the sturdy green, canvas log carrier I wanted from a mail order company. She shows me a plaid flannel shirt, several books, and a ceramic plate. Before it was glazed, she had written on it, "I love you!" in calligraphy.

I had a present for her, a simple silver bracelet I'd bought several months ago in a local crafts shop. I'd had it wrapped and I had hidden it in a drawer under my underwear. I'd totally forgotten about it. She's found the package.

"Is it something for me?" she asks, her eyes glistening. Yes, I flash. She's taking off the wrappings, opening the box. "Oh, I love it," she says. "It's beautiful."

She must go. She can't leave Frances and Charlie any longer. She packs my presents in the log carrier and holds it high for me to see. "You'll be bringing fire wood in with this soon," she says. Yes, yes.

She hesitates in the doorway. "How was Laura?" she asks anxiously. "Was she okay?" Yes, I flash. She was fine.

"Oh, I'm so glad." she says beaming with relief.

Without visitors, time crawls. I try television. It's hard to see without glasses, but to get though the day I watch endless tasteless Christmas specials.

Clare Ann is poised to leave the moment Ingrid arrives. Her belted Navy trench coat, which like the reindeer sweater is her daily uniform, lies across the foot of my bed. She tells me she's heading to Long Island to have Christmas dinner with her sister, her brother-in-law, and their three children. Clare Ann has never been married.

"Do you like roast beef, Robert?" she asks. Yes. "Well that's what we're having—a giant rib roast with baked potatoes. For dessert there'll be plum pudding with hard sauce and ice cream."

She knows I haven't tasted food in weeks. "Do you like your roast beef rare?" she continues. Yes, I adore it that way. "I do too, so my sister always makes sure to keep it extra rare." She smiles cheerfully. I hope you choke on a piece, you sadistic bitch.

It's the first week of January. Dr. Ramsbotham looks grave. I've had my fourth plasmapheresis treatment, and another painful EMG test. It convinced him that the plasmapheresis has had no discernable effect. He's canceling the last one. "There's no point in continuing them, sir." He's so depressed.

The news doesn't surprise me. I didn't think the treatments were working. I hadn't expected them to after hearing that doctor tell his students that plasmapheresis had proved futile for Guillain-Barré in Boston.

Clare Ann thinks I'll recover faster without the treatments. She believes that plasmapheresis has weakened me, slowed my recovery. She could be right. Who knows? The only progress I've made so far is to shake the pneumonia. My eyes are still all I can move.

Old friends, Jean and Harvey Gardner are visiting. The Gardners moved to Nyack when I was in high school and, although they were quite a bit younger, soon became pals of my father and my stepmother. They are also friends of ours.

Jean is English, a war bride. She speaks with the speed of a Gatling gun. Her interests are books and people. Harvey, her husband, is a writer and editor with a dry wit. Like all my visitors, they're made nervous by the respirator.

"Shame about Dick Hanser, wasn't it Rikki?" Jean asks, making light conversation.

"Yes," Rikki says quickly, cutting her off. I'm flashing frantically. I'm demanding to know what happened to him but Rikki ignores me. The Gardners are leaving. I wait.

Finally, we're alone. I want to know about Dick Hanser, my father's best friend. Rikki clutches my hand. "Soon after you got sick we got a call from David saying his father had died suddenly from a heart attack. David thought we might want to go to the funeral. Of course, he hadn't heard about you."

I flash in rage. Tears fill my eyes. How could you keep this from me? You said you told me everything. Goddamnit! What else don't I know? I'm shifting my eyes as fast as I can.

"You're mad at me?" she asks, frightened. Yes, yes. I'm livid, but also devastated, overwhelmed by grief. Silently I weep. Dick was like a wise and gentle uncle. Even when I was very young, he listened to me with interest and respect.

He was an intellectual and an expert on World War II Germany. A fine writer, he was best known as the co-author of "Victory at Sea," the classic television documentary series.

Now I understand why my father's voice has been so grief-ridden. He's lost Dick and I'm certain he thinks I'm dying too. Jesus! My tears gush.

My father and Dick were opposites in many ways. Dick, a minister's son from upstate New York, had a soft, peculiarly precise way of speaking. My father, a Brooklyn boy, was the son of a rough, insensitive man who had spent part of his childhood in an orphanage.

They both started out as newspapermen. Dick went on to be a magazine editor and to win acclaim for his television work. He also wrote books and magazine pieces. My father wrote more than a dozen books and hundreds of magazine articles.

Dick always had a good solid job and paid every bill promptly. My father freelanced. He'd pay the bills when the next check came in. Dick was stodgy; my father is flamboyant. He wrote a successful novel when he was in his early twenties and took all the dough and blew it in Europe. The trip was one of the high points of his life. Dick could have never done that but he admired my father's less regulated life.

On my last visit to Mexico, my father complained to me about Dick. "Hanser is constantly sending me letters and clippings," he bitched.

"What's wrong with that?" I asked, aware that once Dick knew you were interested in a subject, he sent you every printed word he saw about it.

"What's wrong is that he complains that I don't answer him. What does he want me to write, 'The weather is nice here?' The weather's always nice here."

My father had hoped Hanser would visit him in Mexico, but Dick wouldn't go any place that exotic. Bermuda was more his style.

I told my father on that visit that I still admired the opening of his most successful book, "His Eye is on the Sparrow." It's the autobiography of Ethel Waters, the black singer and actress. The book begins:

"I was never a child.

"I never was coddled, or liked, or understood by my family.

"I never felt I belonged.

"I was always an outsider.

"I was born out of wedlock, but that had nothing to do with all this. To people like mine a thing like that just didn't mean much.

"Nobody brought me up.

"I just ran wild as a little girl. I was bad, always a leader of the street gang stealing and general hell raising. By the time I was seven I knew all about sex and life in the raw. I could out curse any stevedore and took sadistic pleasure in shocking people."

"His Eye is on the Sparrow" was an immediate best seller when it was published in 1950.

"That lead is still a classic," I told my father. "After all this time, it hasn't lost any of its punch."

"Hanser gave it to me," he said.

"What do you mean?"

"I had the opening another way. I don't recall now what it was, but it wasn't so direct. Dick suggested I change it. He's always been a superb

editor." It is like him to give Dick all that credit while complaining about having to write him a few lines.

My life has suddenly improved because Clare Ann has taught us a way for me to spell out words. It's simple to do. If I have something to say, I signal with my eyes. Then Rikki asks if the word begins with the first part of the alphabet, A to L. If I don't move my eyes, she knows it's the second part, M to Z. She then calls out the letters. I flash when she hits the right one. We repeat the process for each letter. She writes each one down as we go along so she won't forget.

The first thing I spell is, "I love you." Rikki is so moved she promises she'll save the paper she wrote it on forever. Being able to originate a conversation opens a new world. Why didn't any other health-care professional suggest it?

Clare Ann plans another improvement. She wants me to start sitting-up in a stretcher-chair. It's a contraption that starts out flat, like a stretcher. Then they crank it up to a sitting position. Clare Ann deserves credit for thinking of this.

She needs a doctor's order to start. She asks Dr. Ramsbotham, but he's indecisive, as usual. Dr. Schick thinks it's a splendid idea and quickly gets Dr. Ramsbotham to agree. She says sitting up should help improve my respiration. She's the respiratory doctor. Why didn't she suggest it?

Clare Ann wheels in the stretcher-chair. It's ancient, beat-up, and ugly, like so much of the equipment in this world-famous hospital. Grey vinyl covers its thin pads. "You want to try it now, Robert?" she asks. Yes, I flash. Let's go! I love all movement; any change is fine with me.

"You'll hate it," she predicts.

"Why do you say that?" asks Rikki.

"I don't know why. I just know most people don't like sitting up after they've been lying down for a long time."

I'm different. I'm going to prove her wrong. I'm going to love sitting up. Two nurses are here to help her. They're to slide me from the bed to the chair on the bottom bed sheet. One will cradle my head and the other will shift my legs as Clare Ann pulls the middle of the sheet, the heaviest part. Everyone is tense, and that makes me very nervous.

"His head can snap back. Don't let it slip," Clare Ann warns a young, very frightened nurse. Christ, I'm scared!

"Okay," says Clare Ann. "One, two, three!" She yanks the sheet. My backbone bounces over the crack between the chair and the bed. The respirator tube pulls at my neck. One leg slips off the stretcher-chair. For a moment, I fear it will pull the rest of me to the floor and I'll crash in a heap.

"Goddamnit, watch his leg!" shouts Clare Ann. The nurse assigned to my legs snatches it back. "Jesus, Mary, and Holy Saint Joseph," says Clare Ann.

I'm safe now but please don't ever do this to me again. It's too dangerous. Clare Ann is stuffing pillows around me so I won't slump sideways when she cranks up the chair. She must duck under it to turn the handle. It's a dumb design. The mechanism squeaks as the back slowly rises.

She was right. I hate sitting up. The pain is intense. My backside aches. This thing has no padding at all. It feels as though the bare bones in my buttocks are pressing against bare metal.

Clare Ann is delighted. "You look like a regular person in that chair, Robert," she tells me. I sure don't feel like a regular person. I'm in pain. It's worse than when Laura puts the bed up to feed me.

I'm not actually sitting. I'm reclined, like an astronaut during a blast-off. It feels as though forces many times greater than gravity are grinding me down. I wish I were an astronaut and would soon be weightless. I know my pain will only grow more intense, the pressure greater.

Rikki is back in the room. "It's wonderful to see you sitting up," she says. "You look so much better. Do you like it?" I want to tell her I love it; I want to show Clare Ann she was wrong, but I can't. I'm in too much pain. No, I flash. All I think of is getting back to bed.

"What's wrong?" Rikki wants to know. I rapidly shift my eyes, signaling I want to spell.

"A to L?" she asks, getting out her notebook. No. "M to Z?" Yes.

"M? N? 0? P?" Yes, I signal.

"The first letter is P?" Yes.

"Second letter. "A to L?" Yes.

"A? B?" Yes, yes. You're going too fast!

"Is the second letter B?" No.

"Is it A?" Yes, yes!

"P-A. Is the third letter A to L?" Yes.

"A? B? C? D? E? F? G? H? I?" Yes!

"So far it's "P-A-I, right?" Yes. Why the hell can't you guess the word? Think!

"A to L?" No. Come on, guess!

"M? N?" Yes!

"P-A-I-N, is that it?" Yes! "Oh darling, you're in pain. Do you want to go back to bed?" Yes.

"Bob wants to go back to bed now," Rikki says.

"I know but I want him to stay up a little longer," Clare Ann replies.

"Why?"

"He has to get used to this. He'll be sitting up every day from now on." Oh, Jesus, she hadn't told me that. My life is already hellish, waiting for each hour to pass so she'll turn me. I don't want to give her another way to torment me. No, I signal, no!

"Bob doesn't like that idea," says Rikki.

"It ain't a question of what he likes. I have to do what's best for him."

"But if it causes him pain, is it good?"

"Dr. Schick has ordered that he sit up. She feels it's therapeutic for his respiration and circulation. If you have a problem with that, talk to Dr. Schick."

"Should I call Dr. Schick?" Rikki asks when we're alone. No, I flash. It wouldn't do any good. She'll only back Clare Ann and we'd be marked as uncooperative. Maybe it is important that I sit up—I don't know.

I'm flashing at Rikki. I want to go back to bed now! "Are you in more pain?" she asks. Yes, yes. "When can Bob go back to bed?"

"I'll see if I can find someone to help," Clare Ann says, sauntering slowly out of the room. Oh hurry, please hurry!

"It won't be long," Rikki promises, holding my hand. "The travel agent has been calling about our reservations to Mexico," she says, trying to distract me. "She wants me to send her a check. I think we should cancel." No, I flash angrily.

"Be reasonable," she pleads. "We can always make new reservations." I'm losing track of what she's saying. All my attention is on my aching ass. I must lie down. I can't take the pain any longer. I signal that I want to spell.

She expects a message about the reservations. Instead I spell B-E-D.

"Should I get Clare Ann?" she asks. Yes. Run!

"You want to get back to bed, right Robert?" asks Clare Ann, returning quickly to the room. Yes. She's angry. "This might come as a surprise to you, but you ain't the only one in this hospital. If you think I can get you back in that bed by myself, you're wrong. I need other nurses to help and they're busy right now, so you're just going to have to wait your turn." She whirls around and stalks out.

"I don't know what we can do about her," Rikki despairs. There is no answer— we can't do anything. Clare Ann no longer talks to me, she lectures. We are enemies. What did I do to her?

Ten more terrible minutes and Clare Ann is back.

She sends Rikki away from the room. The two nurses who helped slide me out of bed are going to help get me back. Clare Ann ducks under the chair. This time each turn of the crank lowers my back, every inch down easing the pain. My pleasure is slow and exquisite.

The chair is again a stretcher. I am totally comfortable now, as happy as a man lying on a topless beach in St. Tropez would be. If I was able to roll I'd be worried about falling off, but since I can't move I'm safe. Let me enjoy this for a while.

That can't be. The other nurses must leave. Clare Ann is crawling up on my bed to pull me back because she's not nearly tall enough to reach across it from the other side if she's standing. She looks ridiculous crouched there. If it were someone else, it might look cute or sexy.

I'm scared, although not as scared as I was when they were moving me the other way. The bed is a much wider target than the stretcher-chair. This is a far less dangerous trip.

"One, two, three," says Clare Ann. My spine again bounces over the crack. I sink into the bed. It feels like I'm lying on the finest down. If I hadn't been in the room the whole time, I'd have sworn they'd switched mattresses.

The bed is a mess so Clare Ann is changing the linen, rolling me back and forth. My pleasure is almost great enough to make me forget the pain of the chair. This is ecstasy. Sex for the paralyzed.

Ingrid won't be coming back, Clare Ann tells me the next morning, barely disguising her glee. Ingrid said nothing last night about quitting. She would have told me.

"I ain't kidding," says Clare Ann. "She's gone. She said she couldn't stand working nights any longer." Now what, I wonder. I live at the whim of these nurses. What are we going to do? We'll have to find someone immediately. Go right to the registry and ask for a new nurse, I spell to Rikki as soon as she arrives.

"I'm going to the registry," she tells Clare Ann, who is bringing in new medical supplies. "Bob's very worried about getting someone to work tonight."

"You don't have to," Clare Ann says. "Everything is under control. Robert gets so upset at any change in the nursing schedule. Before you arrived, I was going to tell him that Laura and I have talked it over and, if you agree, we'll split up the work between us. Starting tonight we'll each work twelve-hour shifts. That way you don't need a new nurse. How does that sound?" she asks Rikki.

"It sounds fine to me, but let's ask Bob what he thinks. Would you like that?" she asks me.

Yes, I flash immediately, certain that Clare Ann deliberately put off telling me about Laura to make me worry. She thinks she's teaching me some kind of lesson.

A brief article Clare Ann is reading me from today's *New York Times*, says that Joseph Heller, the author of Catch-22, has Guillain-Barré syndrome. He's in the intensive care unit of an east side hospital, but it gives few details. "So you ain't the only person with Guillain-Barré syndrome," she says, as if I ever thought I was. "I bet Joseph Heller doesn't ask his nurses to turn him all the time." So go take care of Joseph Heller. I give you to him—my gift.

"Did you ever meet Heller?" she asks. No. "Did you read Catch-22?" she wants to know. Yes, I flash. Did you? I spell.

"Yes" she says, and I believe her. She does read, which makes her unusual. She also buys the Times every day.

I keep thinking about Heller and so does she. She's constantly comparing him to me, saying how much better a patient he must be although she knows no more about his situation than I do. For several nights I dream that Heller is my roommate and we spend our time discussing books. Some dream. I can't talk and maybe he can't either.

Late afternoon. Rikki has gone home for the day. "Do that again," says Clare Ann. Do what again? I don't know what she's talking about. "Try moving your jaw. I think you moved it." I try. "You did!"

She drags a floor nurse into the room to see it. "Robert, do it again." She's very excited and strangely proud. It doesn't feel as though my jaw is moving. It's not like when I think I'm moving my hand. Both nurses stare at me.

"I see it!" the other nurse shouts. "His chin moved!"

So, this is how it starts. It's not me imagining things this time. My jaw is actually moving! Other people see it! "A journey of a thousand miles begins with a single step," wrote an ancient Chinese philosopher. I've taken my first step. Nothing can stop me now!

I'm awake through the night, my thoughts racing. My recovery has started at the top of my body, just as the doctors said it would. It will go quickly now.

Clare Ann and I are waiting anxiously for Rikki to arrive so she can see it. I'm thrilled to have good news for her. It's been so long since we've had anything to celebrate.

"We have something to show you," says Clare Ann when Rikki finally gets here. She's turned on every light in the room. "Okay, Robert." Drum roll, please. I give it all I have. "Do you see it?" asks Clare Ann.

Rikki is confused. She doesn't know what she's supposed to look at. "He's moving his jaw," Clare Ann tells her, clearly annoyed.

"Yes, yes, I see it now. Oh, how wonderful! How wonderful!" Rikki cries. Her eyes fill with tears. The moment we're alone, she embraces me. "You're going to make a full recovery. A total recovery," she whispers into my neck over and over, ignoring the respirator tube.

"That's incredible, Bob, incredible," Charlie shouts, leaping around the room when he sees it. His Christmas vacation is nearly over. He's heading back to Maryland tomorrow.

"I'm afraid I see nothing," Dr. Ramsbotham tells us stiffly during his regular afternoon visit. Is he right? Have they all been imagining that I'm moving my jaw?

"Look at his chin," Clare Ann says, barely hiding her anger.

Suddenly he spots it. "Very good, sir, very good! Now, try moving your feet." He lifts the covers, as if he expects to see me twiddling my toes. What kind of an idiot is he? Clare Ann glances at Rikki and Charlie but says nothing. I know she thinks he's a complete fool.

Our friends are wonderful. They make household repairs for Rikki and invite her out on weekends. Rikki has been leaving notes by our back door, telling everyone of my progress. She also tells them that I'm optimistic. I am.

They're playing the Super Bowl tomorrow and Dale Hiestand has asked Rikki if he can come here and watch it with me. How can I say no? Since Dale I will be watching the game, Rikki will stay home, her first day off in the six weeks I've been sick.

After Rikki leaves, Clare Ann tells me she won't be here tomorrow either. I'm frightened. If I had known, I would have asked Rikki to come in but now it's too late. There is no way now to get a message to Rikki. The idea of facing a completely strange daytime nurse alone terrifies me. There is so much more for a day nurse to do and so much more to go wrong.

My fears are groundless, Clare Ann says, but she's wrong. Something bad has happened to me every time she's taken off. The hospital has sent substitutes who knew nothing about respirators and suctioning.

One Jamaican nurse treated me as though I was in a coma. She left me sprawled in horribly uncomfortable positions and didn't respond to my frantic eye signals. Rikki kept asking her to make me more comfortable. The nurse resented that, resented Rikki. To retaliate, she started leaving me off the respirator for much longer periods than necessary when she suctioned me.

Late in the afternoon, Rikki and the nurse got into a shouting match. Rikki told her to leave. She called the registry and told them never to send that woman again. Why doesn't the hospital screen these nurses?

The more I brood, the angrier I get. Clare Ann deliberately waited until after Rikki was gone to tell me she'd also be away. She doesn't want Rikki to help me with the new nurse. She thinks I'm too dependent on Rikki. Too dependent for what?

Laura is so kind. She's doing everything she can to reassure me that I'll be safe. She'll explain everything to the new nurse who is from the Philippines, where she says they have excellent nursing schools. That's why Filipinas are usually good nurses, Laura adds.

Is this true? I don't know. It doesn't help me sleep.

Her name is Rosa. She's a petite, almond-eyed young woman with mocha skin. At first she has trouble understanding my eye signals, but when she catches on, she's quick to help me. She knows about respirators. She's won't accidentally kill me. That's all I should care about.

As the morning passes, things are becoming easier for Rosa. I like her. I don't miss Clare Ann. Rosa has the novel idea that I should be comfortable. She doesn't put my head too high. She has no rule about waiting an hour to turn me and I know she won't force me into the stretcher-chair. Only Clare Ann is ambitious enough to do that.

It would be so wonderful if I could replace Clare Ann with Rosa. I obsess about it. Jesus, I can do it. I can do it tomorrow. I'll just spell it out to Rikki and we'll be rid of Clare Ann. My troubles will be over!

No, I'm learning it's not that simple. Another Filipina nurse has stopped in. Rosa is discussing her young children with her. Because of her children, Rosa is explaining, she only works one or two days a week. She'll never take my case. I must find some other way of getting rid of Clare Ann. There has to be a way.

It's lonely without Rikki. The hours drag. I'm trying to stay awake for Dale. If he found me asleep, he wouldn't disturb me and we'd miss the game. Here he is now. Good to see you, old friend. "Next year we'll watch it at your house," he promises. Yes, I signal but it sounds to me like an impossible dream.

Maybe I have damaged my eyes. Can't tell which team is which. All I see are blurs of colors. Won't worry. Just be happy Dale is here so we can watch together as we have in other years.

But it's not like other years. Dale is spending more time watching my eyes for distress signals than he is looking at the television screen. "I think Bob wants something," he tells Rosa when I flash. Then they try to guess what it is. Each time Rosa turns me, suctions, or catheterizes me, he must leave the room.

The second half has begun and I keep drifting off to sleep. I'm exhausted from worrying all night about the new nurse. Should he leave, Dale keeps asking. No. I don't want

visitors to think I'm easily tired; I don't want them to think
I've changed.

"Well, Robert, I see you survived," Clare Ann says the
next morning. Yeah, I survived, but you almost didn't. If it
weren't for Rosa's children, you'd be on your way.

Each time they move me to the stretcher-chair it scares
me. I also hate sitting in it but Clare Ann is relentless. She
now has me in it, twice a day for up to fifteen minutes at a
time, and she's threatening to lengthen my stays to a half-
hour. She's tried to make it more comfortable by stuffing
pillows under me, but that hasn't helped.

Is something wrong with the chair? It couldn't have
been this hard when it was new. I ask Rikki to squeeze the
pads to see if they have any give. She assures me they do. I
have her sit in it. Is it unusually uncomfortable? It feels all
right to her.

"Why does the chair hurt Bob so much?" Rikki asks.

"It's him. He just don't tolerate discomfort very well,"
Clare Ann says.

"That's not true!" Rikki shouts. "That thing's a torture
chair."

"Torture chair! Torture chair! Don't call it that!" Clare
Ann shouts back. "It's improving his respiration and his
circulation. The doctors want him in it."

"Your wife should appreciate how much work it is
to get you in that chair," Clare Ann tells me bitterly after
Rikki leaves. "There ain't many nurses who would take the
trouble. She should be encouraging you to sit in it longer
instead of helping you watch the clock. Don't you think
so?" I keep my eyes motionless. To disagree would invite
an endless tirade.

"I ain't ever seen a wife like yours. She's in here all the
time. Don't you think she should take more time off? She

could be heading for serious mental problems, you know. I've nursed a lot of sick men and met a lot of wives," she continues, "but I ain't ever met one less helpful than yours."

That fills me with fury. My eyes swing wildly. Don't you criticize Rikki! She's my wife. You don't understand what that means. We've been together for more than twenty years. We've seen the best and the worst of each other. We've raised a child, made a home and had a life. I couldn't have survived one day of this without her.

Clare Ann ignores my frantic eyes. She's like some crazed, self-righteous evangelist. She doesn't let up until the technician comes to check my respirator.

It's late afternoon and Rikki has gone for the day. Dale is visiting. I'm in the chair and the pain is excruciating. Every part of me feels ten times heavier than normal. I signal Dale that I need help and he runs to the nurses' lounge for Clare Ann. "No, you can't go back to bed. Don't bother me again," she says.

"Are you very uncomfortable?" Dale asks after we're alone again. Yes. "You want to lie down?" Yes, God, yes! I'm being conversational; I'm not asking him to get Clare Ann again, but he misunderstands.

She sends Dale from the room. "You'd think you could enjoy your visitor without worrying about your comfort," she says, her voice full of contempt. It's beyond her to imagine my pain. "I'll put you back to bed this time, but don't ever pull this again." She's not doing me any favors. I've been sitting up a long time.

Two nurses are helping. As they slide me from the chair, my head slams into the bedstead making a loud conk. The nurse supporting my head immediately starts apologizing. "Don't worry about it, Mary," says Clare Ann. "It might knock some sense into him."

Dale has left and Clare Ann is starting in about him and my other friends. She claims she's never known anyone to have such terrible friends. They should be more supportive of me, she says. More supportive of her is what she means. I'm lying down, so relieved by being comfortable at last that I don't care what she says.

Before Rikki allows any new visitor in, she tells them what to expect, but no matter what she says they're always stunned. Until now I haven't let Rikki's younger sister, Jinx, and her husband, Howard, see me, but Rikki has talked me into it. They're waiting in the hall now.

Rikki is opening the door. Jinx is rushing to me. She's stroking my face, squeezing my hand, embracing me. Howard stands back against the wall staring, his face pale in shock, clearly horrified by my tubes and respirator. It's so unlike Jinx to cling to me. In all the years I've known her she's never kissed or touched me. That's not her style. I greet women I barely know with hugs and kisses, but I've never even given Jinx a peck on the cheek.

I first met her, a dark-haired version of Rikki, on her sixteenth birthday, soon after Rikki and I started dating. I was a cub reporter on the White Plains newspaper, and Rikki had a temporary job there as secretary to the editor. Jinx had come to the city room that day so Rikki, who is five years older, could take her to apply for her driver's license and to a birthday lunch.

I've cared for Jinx for a long time. I've watched her grow up, graduate from high school and college and become a potter. She brought Howard, who is a fine cabinetmaker, to meet us soon after they began living together. We were at their wedding. We love her children. I couldn't like Howard, a shy, intelligent man, more if I had chosen him myself, but Jinx has always been physically distant. There is no distance between us today, only love.

Sometimes, in moments of despair, I'll doubt if there are any decent people in the world. Then I'll remember Jinx and Howard and their kids in their farmhouse in rural Massachusetts and know there are.

Here we go again. Dr. Schick wants me to try a new, super comfortable bed. It works, she says, something like a waterbed. Instead of water, the mattress is filled with bits of plastic which are kept suspended by air from a powerful fan.

The bed supposedly prevents bedsores. Since they are a result of poor nursing care, Clare Ann regards this bed as a personal insult. What's more, she believes, it's my fault the bed is being forced on us. Dr. Schick wants to order it, she claims, because of my constant complaints about being uncomfortable.

I don't argue, but the bed isn't my fault. Ingrid asked for it after the swinging bed fiasco. Her concern for my comfort was always secondary. She thought it would save her the work of turning me so often. She had no trouble selling Dr. Schick the idea. She seems drawn to mechanical beds of every imaginable description. I wonder what she sleeps on.

I have been against the bed until I learn that Clare Ann won't be able to get me out of it and into the stretcher-chair. Now, I can't wait to try it.

The bed has arrived. Trumpets please. It's such a big, blocky thing that it takes three nurses just to push it into the room. Dr. Schick has come to watch. Before I know it, they're raising my hospital bed way up to make it level with the new bed. Now they're sliding me over. Hey, wait a minute! This thing is hard as asphalt. Is this some kind of a joke?

"I'll turn it on," says one of the nurses who seems to be the authority on it. She clicks a switch and the lights of my room flicker as a powerful fan starts whooshing. The mattress, hissing like a cobra, turns liquidy soft.

"The bed makes it much easier to turn the patient," explains the nurse who flicked the switch. She gives me a gentle shove and I roll slowly from my right to my left side in the cloud-like softness. Whee! It's fun! "You have to immobilize the patient to wash or catheterize him," she says, stopping the motor. I'm immediately frozen like a statue.

"You'll want him sitting up when you feed him," she continues, hitting the switch and making me fluid once more. The lights dim again. This thing must suck up more juice than an electric chair.

"Unfortunately," the nurse goes on, "there's no way to mechanically raise the head of this bed so we have to get him to sit up." How the hell will you do that, I wonder.

"He can't move at all," Clare Ann explains.

"In that case, you'll need help," the other nurse says but before she can describe it, I need suctioning. That's not so simple now. When Clare Ann tries to stick the catheter into my trach, I drift out of position. It's like someone trying to thread a moving needle. Finally, they turn off the motor stopping me.

It will take three nurses to sit me up. Two of them pull my shoulders and arms while a third shoves an aqua-colored foam backrest behind me. It make me much more erect than I ever am in the stretcher-chair.

Nothing supports me. I slump forward. Drool and mucous run off my chin and over my hospital gown. I'm going to be sitting like this for a half-hour or more each time I'm fed, I suddenly realize. The pain is horrendous. Even the stretcher-chair isn't this bad.

"You don't care for this much, do you Robert?" Clare Ann asks cheerfully, packing pillows around my neck to support my head. No, I flash, knowing she thinks I'm getting just what I deserve.

"Why doesn't he like it?" Dr. Schick wants to know.

"Robert ain't big on sitting up," Clare Ann tells her. She's connected my nose tube to the feeding tube and dumped a can of nutrient into the plastic sack at its end. The tube turns white as the stuff starts its journey to my stomach.

"Are you comfortable?" Rikki asks when she's finally allowed into the room. It's agony sitting up, I let her know.

That's difficult for her to understand. She squeezes the foam backrest. It feels soft to her. "Do you like the bed itself?" Yes, I flash, but I don't yet know if I do. I want the feeding over so I can lie down again and try it.

~

This is my second day in the bed, and both Clare Ann and I realize it is a mistake. As far as I'm concerned, the torture of having to sit up totally offsets the slight gain in comfort. The bed is nothing but trouble for Clare Ann. It's so high that to reach me, she has to stand on a shaky stool. The heat from the motor, which runs almost constantly, has turned the room into a sauna. It's forcing her to work without her beloved reindeer sweater.

Despite all this, she refuses to criticize the bed. She's teaching me a lesson. She thinks I somehow demanded to get this bed and therefore she's going to force me to lie in it.

I've complained to Dr. Ramsbotham, but he says I should give it more time. More time! What good will that do? He doesn't understand the problem—any problem.

~

I haven't seen Dr. Schick since they delivered the bed or

I'd ask her why she's allowing me to forego the stretcher-chair. I thought she believed that it's vital to my survival.

Another major bed crisis. "Jesus, Mary and Holy St. Joseph," says Clare Ann, rapidly clicking the on/off switch. Zilch. Now what? She's checking to see if the bed is still plugged in. There are no loose wires or anything else obviously wrong.

It's probably only a broken switch, I think, not that I'm making any suggestions. I'm enjoying myself enormously. Oh, boy, another mechanical bed may have died.

Clare Ann is out at the nurses' station, trying to reach someone from maintenance. That's going to be tough on a Saturday. If they're not able to fix it, they'll have to get me a regular bed. I hope it doesn't take long. This deflated pile of plastic junk is incredibly hard.

"Maintenance says they ain't coming for three or four hours cause they got a busted pipe in another building," she reports. She's steaming and I panic. Three or four hours! I can't last another ten minutes! I'm swinging my eyes to get her attention. You can't leave me here!

"You worrying about your own comfort again, Robert?" she taunts. "If you didn't have everyone so concerned about making you comfortable, you wouldn't be in this bed to begin with. I ain't going to be able to reach the doctors today," she says. So then what? I stay here forever? She's out of the room again. Jesus, don't desert me! Please, please, Clare Ann!

Minutes pass. Now she's back with a gang of nurses and an ordinary hospital bed. They've sliding me over. I'm saved! "Tomorrow," she warns meanly, trying to take away my pleasure, "you go back in the stretcher-chair." I don't care. That's tomorrow. If I'm lucky, she'll be hit by a truck.

I've been back in a regular hospital bed several days now and life has returned to normal, if you can call anything about this normal.

Rikki is happy because she sees I'm getting better. "Do you love me?" she asks playfully when we're alone. Yes, yes, I flash.

"Do you love me more than ever?" Yes, yes, yes! I'm making a joke of it by using everything I have to answer. I'm moving my eyes, my jaw, and my head side-to-side (a recent improvement) a tiny bit. Her eyes glisten, knowing what effort this takes.

"You'll never be able to tell me you love me more beautifully than this," she cries, burying her face in the pillow near my head. God, do I love her!

Dr. Stone, the head of rehabilitation medicine for the hospital, has told Rikki that once I'm off the respirator it will be best for me to finish my recovery at a rehabilitation hospital. He predicts I'll eventually move from a wheelchair to a walker, to crutches, a cane, then, hopefully, nothing at all. It sounds slow but any talk of progress cheers me.

Though he had said it's too early for me to start physical therapy, he said, Clare Ann's argues with him and he changes his mind. Now every weekday afternoon Lindy, a therapist who exercises my arms and legs by moving and stretching them—it's called passive range of motion —visits my room.

Lindy is a delight, a preppie little blonde who wears starched, button-down blue shirts from Brooks Brothers. She's very careful not to hurt me.

"Stretch him more," Clare Ann urges. Lindy thinks Clare Ann is joking but I know she's not. She honestly believes the more I suffer the faster I will heal. Considering what I've been through, if she were right I'd be tap dancing by now.

Hooray! My lungs have improved. Dr. Schick is adjusting the respirator to give me larger breaths. With the new settings, I first feel as though I'm gasping my last, but by the time Laura starts her shift, I've adjusted.

"Are you all right?" Laura asks, her nose twitching like crazy. Yes, I flash, I feel fine. Why is she studying me so intently? Your fingernails look blue, she says. Come on Laura, it's the middle of the damn night. Let me go to sleep. Now, she's got some resident with a bad complexion here and he's drawing blood to check my oxygen level. Come on!

Oh, Jesus, they've found something bad! They've been whispering and now they're calling for a chest x-ray. What the hell could it be? More pneumonia, or is it lung cancer?

It must be serious. It's barely dawn and they've got Dr. Schick in here. She's explaining that I've torn a lung. She must have caused it by hiking the respirator settings, but she doesn't tell me that. She must think I'm an idiot. No wonder everyone is suing doctors.

This is a minor setback, don't worry, she says, but she looks worried. Could I die? I ask. She's evasive. If my chest cavity starts filling with fluid, she explains, I'll need tubes to drain it. To put them in, they'll actually punch holes between my ribs. Clare Ann, who has just come on duty, claims it won't hurt a bit. Sure, and I'll be playing volleyball this afternoon.

Rikki's here early. They phoned and told her there was a problem. She's trying so hard not to look concerned but I can see she's scared. Am I in any pain, she asks. No, I tell her honestly. She hasn't noticed the ominous looking cardboard cartons in the corner. No one's told her that the tubes are in them or about the fluid that could block my lungs and kill me. I wonder how they will know if it suddenly happens. Every time I seem to be making progress, something bad happens.

Clare Ann is still trying to sell me on the idea that having chest tubes pushed through your ribs is almost fun. It's such a minor procedure, she says, so trivial, that any resident can do it. Jesus, I don't want those things in me. Not more tubes keeping me alive. I don't want the pain!

~

Because of the lung tear, I'm back to twice-a-day chest x-rays. What's all this radiation doing to me? Will it give me cancer someday? What nonsense, Clare Ann says. Why worry about a few chest x-rays? Cumulative damage, I want to tell her, and I manage to spell out C-U-M-U-L-A-T-I-V-E. She stares at me as if I've gone mad. But the next day, while I'm in the damn stretcher-chair, she reads me a *New York Times* article that warns of the cumulative affects of x-rays. She's amazed that I knew something she didn't.

It's been a week since my lung was torn. Dr. Schick says it has already healed. I'll believe her when they take their scary chest tube boxes out of my room.

Now that I've dodged that bullet, Clare Ann has planned another assault on my body. She's convinced the doctors that I need a gastrectomy. It means putting a feeding tube directly though my abdomen, into my stomach. No way, I tell her. You'll be more comfortable without a nose tube, she argues. That tube is no problem for me. It's a problem for her and the other nurses because it gets clogged with the liquid vitamin C they feed me. This won't happen with the stomach tube because it is larger, she says.

No, I tell her.

I'm selfish, she says. I don't care about nurses' problems. Nobody respects nurses, she adds. Even supermarket checkout clerks have higher starting salaries. She brings this up all the time, as if I'm responsible. She's getting $150 a shift. That's more than any supermarket clerk I ever heard of.

Why not have the operation, she keeps asking. I don't want the scars, I stupidly tell her.

"You think your body is beautiful?" she asks, laughing scornfully. Jesus, I don't even like my body, but I don't want to wind up a freak. I already have a hole in my neck. I don't need a matching one in my stomach.

Clare Ann brings in Dr. Schick to help make the sale. "The scar will be very small, hardly noticeable," she purrs. I'll bet there are no scars on her sleek bod.

"You might even start swallowing sooner without that tube blocking your throat," she adds, almost as an afterthought. "The tube could be inhibiting your swallowing reflex. The sooner it returns, the sooner you'll eat normally again."

That's the first good argument I've heard for the operation. "Will you think it over?" she asks. Yes, I promise.

Every evening after Laura arrives she spends a half-hour or more in the nurses' lounge with Clare Ann. They go over the details of my day, from Clare Ann's point of view of course. I always try to guess what they discussed. Tonight, Clare Ann's been pushing Laura again to sell me on the tube.

"If you have the operation," Laura says, "you won't have to sit up so long when you're fed because the food will go in much faster." That's advantage number two. I'm weakening. All day I've been imagining eating real food again.

I'd much rather say yes to Laura than to Clare Ann or Dr. Schick. If I'm changing my mind, I should change it now. Okay, I suddenly tell her, let them do it. "Are you serious?" she asks joyously. She'll get big points from Clare Ann for this. Yes, I'm serious.

"Congratulations, Robert, you finally came to your senses!" says Clare Ann at the start of her shift. Soon I'm visited by Dr. Clark. He's a surgeon out of central casting, graying, handsome and deep-voiced. He, as they say, inspires confidence. It's a minor procedure, no anesthesia, he assures me. I'll be back in my room in no time. Have dinner ready, please.

The food commercials on television are really driving me crazy now. Burger King has a series asking, "Aren't you hungry?" I want to shout back, "Are you kidding?" Its burgers look to me like *haute cuisine*. Bring on the surgeons!

Then there is Red Lobster. This ad features a tight shot of a steamy, red lobster being cracked open. A fork pulls out the succulent meat and dips it in warm butter. This really kills me. When I'm able to eat, I want a lobster, I tell Laura. She promises she'll bring me one then. She means it too, but I doubt she'll remember.

The operation was supposed to be at eleven this morning. Clare Ann says surgeons are always late and so far she's right. Hours slip by. I want it over. Rikki is restless. She has things to do at home. Finally, she asks would I mind if she left. No, I tell her, but I don't want her to go. If she's not here I'm afraid something terrible will happen to me.

"When they take you to the operating room, try to notice the nice, old-fashioned hallway," Rikki says, kissing me goodbye. I smile to myself. When we travel she's always pointing out things I might miss. She's still doing it.

"He ain't going to have much of a chance to look at the decor," Clare Ann says, disgustedly. She thinks we're ninnies.

It's past five in the afternoon. Clare Ann has called to find out what's holding things up. "Maybe they'll postpone the operation until tomorrow," she says just as they come for me.

I don't see Dr. Clark in this group of Asians in green scrubs and puffy hats. They look more like stir-fry cooks than surgeons. Where is Dr. Clark? I contracted with him for this job.

They've detached the respirator and one of them squeezes an ambu bag at my neck. They're rolling me through the hall. Sorry Rikki, I can't see anything but an off-white ceiling. We're on an elevator now, through a corridor and into an operating room. Still no Dr. Clark!

They've hooked me to another respirator and rigged a sheet to block my view. I can't watch the operating room drama. I can't see a damn thing except one Asian doctor. The operating table is torturously uncomfortable. Think of something else.

They're poking my belly. Laura shaved it last night. Never saw anyone so nervous with a disposable razor. I'm glad she wasn't doing my pubic area.

Clare Ann shaves my face with my old Norelco. I had put it away for Charlie ages ago when I went back to using a blade. Guess Rikki didn't know about that because when Clare Ann asked for a razor, she brought it in. Clare Ann scrubs my face with it as hard as she can, yanking off the whiskers. A light, circular motion works best, but that's not her style.

They're injecting my stomach with something to deaden the pain. It doesn't help make this table feel more comfortable. Drill the hole or whatever you do, just do it! Get it over!

The doctors are discussing something but I can't make out what they're saying. "Just take it easy, Mr. Samuels," says the one nearest me. Oh my God, what's happening? Something is wrong! Rikki, you should have stayed. I should have insisted. I feel myself slipping away in helpless terror— the light is dimming, going from grey to black.

"You awake, now?" Laura asks anxiously. Yes. I'm back in my room. Her big white teeth and soft brown eyes are coming into focus. Her nose is twitching inches from mine. Everything is hazy and painful.

"Do you remember what happened?" No.

"When they examined your stomach," she explains, "they found you had a hernia. They had to put you under to repair it. They must have told you." No. "Well, it's over now. You have the stomach tube and your hernia is fixed," she says.

Breathing hurts. I fear I will rip my stitches open with each breath from the respirator. Maybe they can set it to give me shallower breaths.

"Did you know you had a hernia?" Laura asks. Yes. "Did you ever see a doctor about it?" No. "You knew you had a hernia and you never saw a doctor?" Yes. She's incredulous. She'd have run to a doctor.

I first noticed the lump over my navel a couple of years ago. I'd guessed it was a hernia but since it only hurt if I stretched hard, I ignored it. I was afraid a doctor would recommend an operation. I didn't want any part of that. Well, now it's done.

Laura has a habit that hadn't bothered me before, but now it is causing me agony. Each time she finishes suctioning me, she pushes a button on the machine to give me an extra big breath. She's the only nurse who does this and she does it frequently because she's a worrier and suctions me so often. It was mildly annoying before the operation, but now the extra air is stretching my stomach against the stitches. It is screamingly painful.

No! I flash each time she pushes the button but she doesn't understand what's wrong. She wouldn't unnecessarily hurt me.

"Very clever, Robert," Clare Ann says the next morning, lifting the sheet and peering at my stomach. "You got two operations for the price of one." For a change, I'm glad to see her because she never touches the big breath button. I wonder if she would if she knew how much pain it gives me.

I'm flashing. I want to tell her I'm thirsty. "What do you want now?" she asks. "Suctioning?" No.

"You can't want to be turned again?" No. Don't want turning today. It would hurt like hell. "Well then what?" she asks, impatiently. "Spell it." She hates waiting for me to spell. I'm parched. I haven't been this dry since the summer Rikki and I toured Morocco in an unairconditioned car. T-H-I-R-S-T-Y, I tell her.

"That's from the anesthesia," she explains. "You'd love a glass of water, wouldn't you?" Yes, yes! I could drink a gallon. "Well, you can't have any. You can't swallow," she reminds me. I flash in protest. I'm dying of thirst!

"When the doctor comes, I'll ask if I can put some ice in your mouth." W-H-E-N? "I don't know. Maybe soon." Water! Dump a bucket of ice water in my mouth!

What do you know, here comes Dr. Clark, the surgeon. I never expected to see him again. "What's wrong?" he asks Clare Ann, when he sees my rapidly shifting eyes.

"The anesthesia has made Robert very thirsty."

"You can give him some ice to suck," he suggests, not realizing I can't suck. That doesn't matter. Just put the ice in my mouth now! I want it now! I'm moving my eyes so quickly the room spins.

My stomach tube is in top-notch shape, he tells us after examining me. Where were you yesterday, I'd like to ask. "Two operations for the price of one," he chuckles, looking at my hernia. I'll bet he charges for both. Ice, I want ice. He'll take the stitches out in a few days. I don't give a damn. Ice! Give me ice!

"Your lack of patience embarrasses me," Clare Ann says when he leaves. "Do you think I have an ice machine in the room?"

It's a rhetorical question. Naturally, I don't answer. "Do you?" she repeats. Uh, oh, she wants an answer—she's insisting on it. No, I signal. I know there's no ice machine in the room. She's always acting like a schoolteacher.

She goes for the ice. The machine couldn't be far since she's back so quickly. She's putting some in my mouth. It feels great. I can't even move it around with my tongue. Still, it's incredibly refreshing.

"This is a mess," says Clare Ann, after a couple of minutes. "Your pillow is soaked!" I can't swallow so what did she expect? The ice is melting and water is dribbling out of my mouth. There is no place else for the water to go. The bed has to get wet. But so what? Who cares? She cares. She gets towels to cover the damp pillowcase.

Rikki is here and Clare Ann's telling her about the hernia. "Would you like to see the stitches and the tube?" Of course Rikki would. She loves grisly sights.

No more ice for me, Clare Ann decides. It's too messy. Instead, she shows Rikki how to dribble drops of ice water from a clean washcloth to my mouth. "Just a little at a time," she cautions before leaving us.

I'm flashing for more water. A couple of drops can't possibly satisfy me. "Is this enough?" Rikki asks. No. Dump the whole damn basin in my mouth. She squeezes the washcloth harder. "I'm so glad there's something I can do for you." Yes.

Clare Ann barges in. "The towel and pillow slip are soaked!" she cries. She's nearly hysterical. "I'll have to change it." So what? It's unavoidable. "Mrs. Samuels, will you please leave us." What's the big deal? She changes my linen all the time anyway.

"Can't your wife follow simple instructions?" she asks. "I tell her to give you a few drops and she floods the bed. I have to change the whole thing." Leave it. I don't mind.

She's hurting me! She's rolling me back and forth, as if

I didn't have stitches. She's crazy, furious. I'm afraid she'll yank the tube out of my stomach! Oh, Clare Ann, the bed isn't that wet.

"You begged for more water, didn't you Robert?" Ignore the question. Don't answer. Pretend you're a prisoner of war. "Well, didn't you?" she persists, her green eyes bright with anger. "You did, didn't you? That's right, ain't it?" No, I finally lie, trying to end her tirade.

"You're telling me she gave it to you without your asking? She poured water in your mouth for no reason? Is that it, Robert?" Her lips are curled in contempt. I WILL NOT ANSWER, YOU BITCH!

I'm saved. Her friend, a male nurse, has come to take her to lunch. They're going to the local pizza joint, she tells me. "How does that sound to you, Robert?" she asks meanly. Fine and dandy! If you don't mind, bring me back a slice and a beer. No, on second thought, hold the pizza. I'll just have the beer.

Rikki is back. The room is once again in order. The bed has been remade and a fresh towel covers the pillow. None of that matters to me. My stitches hurt and I'm parched. All I want is water.

"Only a few drops, a very few drops this time," Clare Ann warns as she gets ready to go. "More water could be dangerous. Robert could drown." That's absurd. How could I drown? It couldn't happen. There's a balloon device on the trach tube, making it impossible for water from my mouth to reach my lungs.

Rikki's doling out the water drop by drop. I'm flashing in frustration. That's not enough! "You want more?" Yes. She squeezes out a couple of additional drops. More! "I can't give you more," she pleads. "It's dangerous." No. "But Clare Ann said you could drown!" No, no.

"You don't believe her?" No. "You think she's lying?" I shift my eyes back and forth, meaning I don't know why she said it. "Are you certain that it won't hurt you?" Yes. Gradually, she's letting me have more.

Clare Ann's hand immediately goes to my pillow when she returns. "You soaked it again," she tells Rikki. "I don't know why you can't follow instructions." I'm filled with dread as she asks Rikki to leave.

"Jesus, Mary, and Holy Saint Joseph!" she explodes as the door closes. "What's wrong with your wife? Does she want to drown you?" The witness doesn't have to answer. "Is that why she flooded the bed?"

She's rolling me over to get the damp sheet from under me. I want to scream in pain. I'm sure she's ripping out my stitches and the tube. "I'll be at lunch," Rikki calls through the door.

I'm defenseless now. "You are the worst patient, the most demanding, I've had in all my years of nursing," she says. At least I have some distinction, I joke to myself, but it's not funny. I'm hurt and scared.

Is it my fault? Do I expect too much from her? Isn't she supposed to help make my life easier? No other nurse has complained about me. Laura doesn't think I'm terrible.

"You are completely selfish," she continues. "You don't care how many times I change the bed as long as you get your ice." You don't understand how thirsty I am, I want to tell her.

"You care only about your own comfort. I carefully position you but you get your wife to move your leg." I want to tell her it's because she bends my leg too much. Christ, she even uses icy sand bags to hold it in place. I only ask Rikki to move it when it's painfully cramped. I try to avoid trouble. I don't want her angry with me all the time; I don't want to fight. I want to get well and leave.

"I've explained over and over that you're positioned in a specific way for a specific reason," she rages. "That's why it's important you not be moved. You and your wife ain't capable of understanding my reasons. You lack the scientific training."

Oh, come on Clare Ann! It doesn't take a nuclear physicist to know that you position me to avoid bedsores and to keep my feet from permanently pointing down. Unlike you, the other nurses also try to make me comfortable. Laura always asks if I'm okay after she turns me. Even Ingrid wanted me to be comfortable.

I'm so sick of you and this whole damn business. I want to get up and walk out of here and onto the beach in Puerto Vallarta and never see you again. I want to sit with my father at a sidewalk cafe in Cuernavaca and talk books and baseball. What would he think of Clare Ann? Jesus, if he didn't know how she treats me he'd think she's terrific. He loves the Irish and people from Brooklyn.

"Do you want to get better, Robert?" Don't answer. You don't have to answer that. "Do you?" she insists, pausing dramatically. "I don't think you do," she says at last when she realizes I'm not going to respond. "You enjoy being waited on hand and foot."

I'm alone with Rikki now. Tears stream down my face. I can't control myself. "What's wrong, darling? What's wrong?" she asks. I didn't want her to see me crying. It will only make her miserable. There's nothing she can do to change things anyway. "Tell me what's wrong?" she pleads.

I H-A-T-E C-L-A R-E A-N-N, I finally spell.

"Did she hurt you?"

C-O-N-S-T-A-N-T H-U-M-I-L-I-A-T-I-N-G L-E-C-T-U-R-E-S.

"I know. I sometimes hear her through the door. I can't

understand her words but I hear the tone. It sounds like she's repeating the same thing over and over."

H-A-T-E H-E-R, I sob.

"I can call the registry and tell them to send someone else." No, I flash. They won't find anyone good who will come regularly. I'll wind up with a different nurse every day.

Rikki has asked other nurses to work for us, but when they learn they'll be replacing Clare Ann they immediately lose interest. They're all afraid of her. No one will step on her turf.

There's another problem too. Laura says she'll quit if we fire Clare Ann. I should realize, she tells me, that Clare Ann is the best nurse in the entire hospital and I'm lucky to have her. If I don't have the sense to keep Clare Ann, she won't work for me.

When I complain to Laura about Clare Ann she says I must be exaggerating. If she allowed herself to believe me, she would have to do something. It is the same problem sexually abused children often have when they ask their parents for help: "He's the best uncle in the whole world, so shut up."

Despite that, I'm happy with Laura. She's cheerful, kind and competent. If she were on duty 24 hours a day, my only problem would be recovering. When she's here, I actually enjoy myself. If I could laugh, I'd be laughing with her much of the time. She's funny about television, which she finds generally moronic. It's hard to argue with that. Because she doesn't own a set, she sees TV with a fresh eye.

The eleven o'clock news, with its bland Kens and Barbies reciting tales of rape, murder, and general mayhem, earns her full scorn. "Is this news?" she'll ask after another report on the 380-pound New Jersey rapist. I don't tell her that I've covered scores of similar stories.

~

This morning, when Laura takes the pillow from under my head and lowers the top of the bed to wash my hair, I turn my head side-to-side for the first time. It's so liberating, like being in a swing. I'm in control. I can stop at various points and start it going again at will. I tease her by pretending my neck is stuck.

I also can shrug now when I'm indifferent and grit my teeth when I'm angry. Rikki finds it side-splittingly funny when I grit them at Clare Ann when she turns her back.

I'm allowing many more visitors. Everyone's welcome except for people from Texaco. I'm still afraid that if they see me they'll think I'll never be able to come back to work.

Some friends are close to tears when they first see me. They feel sorrier for me than I feel for myself. A few have told Rikki that after they visit, they lie in bed at night pretending they can't move, trying to experience what I'm going through. Others have had nightmares about being paralyzed.

They're a verbal bunch so they assume being mute must be the worst part. They're wrong. Not being able to move is the worst part. If I could just roll over when I want and make myself comfortable, I wouldn't mind not speaking for a few months.

Some of them seem desperate to make it easier for me to communicate. They just want to do something. Bob Cone, an inventor of photo chemicals, and Ted Merrill, a journalist, think that if I learned Morse Code, I'd be able to talk by clicking my teeth. I find the idea ludicrous, but they are serious. They've sent me a cassette of Morse Code lessons for beginners. After a couple of minutes of listening,

I plead with Rikki to shut it off. The dots and dashes are driving me crazy.

Fred Burrell has another idea. He's been working feverishly in his photo studio, building what he calls, "a talking machine." He's written phrases on three clear, acrylic wheels and attached them to a six-foot long acrylic strip. He says Rikki can turn the wheels so that the phrases form sentences. We don't want to hurt Fred's feelings so we don't say it's far simpler for me to spell things out.

The contraption stands in a corner of the room, an object of fascination for my bored medical students. They seem much more interested in it than they are in me. Sometimes, unexpectedly, Fred's talking machine rolls silently from its corner and topples to the floor with a terrifying crash. To my delight, it happened today while Dr. Ramsbotham was asking me to move my toes. "Oh, my! Oh, my!" he cried, jumping into the air.

Rikki has surprised me with two large albums of all our old pictures and snapshots. She has begun with baby pictures of both of us and ended with recent vacations. The pictures bring a rush of memories and emotions.

There we are getting married. We're so young! We were both in our early twenties. God, we look like kids! Babies, that's what we were, babies. It wasn't long before we had our own baby.

Now, countless pictures of Charlie. What a happy little person he was. So small! Here's a birthday party. He must have been three or four. Just look at my father! He certainly wasn't frail then. Oh, I forgot that we had that nice picture of my stepmother Louise with Joan. Everyone's so young. It wasn't that long ago. Yes, it was. It was almost twenty years ago.

My father was middle-aged then. Now he's old, Joan's gone and Charlie is almost an adult. Rikki and I are in our middle years. These are facts. It doesn't matter that I don't feel any older—I am older and so is everyone else.

I have no big regrets. I've traveled, done some good work and known some wonderful people. I've had my share of fun and love. I've been a good son, husband and father. I know I have. Is that enough? I don't know.

"Is that all there is?" asks a brittle Peggy Lee after a long ride on a bumpy road. I understand what she's saying but I want to shake her and ask, "Is that all there is compared to what?"

My father raised me to think it a privilege to be alive. I try to treasure every experience, every sunset, but I often don't even notice. That's so sad. Time flees.

Rikki and I emptied Joan's apartment after she died. I kept thinking what if it is all a terrible mistake and she's still alive? She'll never forgive us for getting rid of her things. How could I explain? But she was dead. She wasn't coming back.

The objects that had meant so much to her life—her pictures, her high school year book and love letters—meant nothing to us. We pitched them all out. A life gone. The death rattle her vacation slides made fluttering against the metal incinerator shaft still haunts me. Someday someone will throw our pictures away too. That hadn't occurred to me until we cleared out my sister's apartment.

For months after Joan's death, I would wake suddenly in the middle of the night, terrified by the absolute certainty of my own eventual death. This no longer happens. I've adjusted; I guess its part of getting older.

"Who knows where the time goes?" a wistful Judy Collins wonders. It just goes, your time just goes and here I am on this fucking respirator, unable to stir, unable to talk and my life is slipping by. The picture albums make that clear.

Tears pour down my face. Rikki dabs at them with paper tissue. "We had so many good times," she cries through her own tears, "and we'll have so many more. You'll make a full recovery. You're going to make a full recovery!" Yes, yes, I flash. Yes!

She's about to leave. I signal that I want to spell. I L-O-V-E Y-O-U V-E-R-Y M-U-C-H, I tell her.

Then she's gone. Everyone gets to leave, but I'm here twenty-four hours a day, seven days a week. That's the terrible loneliness of illness. There should be relief patients just as there are relief nurses. When do I resume my normal life? This patient is burned out! Phone down to the bullpen and warm up someone else!

They're going to try testing my vital capacity again. That's a measure of how much air I can inhale and exhale on my own. The results were zero a month ago, but Clare Ann has asked them to try again. She thinks I've improved. She's been encouraging me to attempt a few breaths on my own each time she suctions me. She's much more impatient for me to recover than any doctor. She looks for improvement, pushes for it. It's as though she feels my slowness reflects badly on her.

I'm sitting up in the damn chair, surrounded by dozens of photographs that Rikki has taped to the walls. Shaun, the respiratory technician, is here to test me. Clare Ann has no authority over him, but she orders him around like an incompetent servant. He's a big, good-looking, puppy-dog of a kid in his early twenties. He's much too polite to stand up to her.

She gives him a hard time every time he comes to change the hoses. She pretends it's friendly kidding, but there's a sharp, hostile edge. She's always pleasant to the other technicians, all of whom are older and more self-confident.

When we're alone Shaun calls her Nurse Ratched, after the sadistic character the actress Louise Fletcher made famous. Shaun is the only person I've run across in this hospital who hasn't told me how wonderful Clare Ann is.

Everything is ready for the test. Shaun has the measuring device in my mouth while Clare Ann squeezes my lips around it to stop air from leaking. "Now, breathe in!" he shouts. I give it my all. "Blow out, blow out! Push!" I think I'm breathing but I can't tell. I thought I was the last time.

"Well?" asks Clare Ann.

"Again!" orders Shaun, ignoring her. I do it. I try another time. "Once again!" I'm exhausted, totally out of air.

He quickly reconnects the hose and removes the instrument from my mouth. My lungs inflate and my chest swells. Relief!

"Well, anything?" Clare Ann asks.

"Yes," he smiles, "350 cc's."

"Very nice, Robert, very nice," she says. Very nice, indeed! I'm ecstatic! I am on my way to a complete recovery!

It's a big step, Dr. Schick says, but I'll have to wait until I reach 1,000 cc's before they'll start weaning me off the machine. There's no telling how long it will take. It could come fast. She can't guess but she's encouraged. So am I.

There are other hopeful signs. They no longer need to catheterize me. To attract attention, I can make a clicking sound by putting my tongue against my teeth sucking in air. It's loud enough for nurses in the hall to hear. I'm also moving my arms a bit above the elbow.

Rikki has started visiting rehabilitation hospitals to find the best one. She met a woman with Guillain-Barré at one. She had come to the rehab hospital on a stretcher by ambulance. Now, six-months later, she's on crutches. They're discharging her and expect her to make a complete recovery.

That's soon going to be my story. All I have to do to get out of here is to breathe without a respirator.

I thought spring had begun, but this morning I wake to a raging blizzard. It's so bad out that even Clare Ann is a half-hour late. "Your wife won't make it today, Robert," she tells me gleefully. I'm sure she's right. The television stations keep interrupting themselves with fresh storm bulletins. Except for Super Bowl Sunday, it will be the first day Rikki has missed.

"There won't be anyone here to move your leg," Clare Ann taunts when she's ready to go to lunch, but she's wrong. Rikki is coming through the door like the cavalry in a John Wayne movie. No blizzard can stop her!

~

"Starting tomorrow I'm taking three days off," Clare Ann says casually a few days later, just before she's ready to turn me over to Laura. "I already let the registry know. I'm sure they'll send you a good nurse." I'm boiling with rage and fear. If she'd told me sooner, I would have had Rikki come in early to make sure the new nurse knows what she is doing.

Did you know that Clare Ann was taking off? I ask Laura as soon as I see her.

"Yes, I did."

Why didn't you tell me?

"It was up to Clare Ann to tell you," she says. "I didn't want to interfere." There is no point in being angry with Laura. She's afraid of Clare Ann just like everyone in this hospital, including me.

I'm learning that a nurse named Kathleen Cunningham will fill in. That supposedly is good news. Laura says Kathleen knows respirators and is excellent. We're waiting. Laura has bathed me and straightened the room in anticipation of the new nurse. Finally, she's here. "Hi there," she says with a soft Irish brogue.

"Do you need anything now?"

No.

"I'll be back after I talk with Laura," she promises. Clare Ann never asks if I need anything. Before I can start fretting about how long she'll be out of the room, she's back.

"I'll bet you were really worried about who was going to come through that door this morning," she says.

Yes.

"Well, I don't blame you. It must be terrible to lie there wondering what strange creature the registry will send this time."

Kathleen Cunningham is the complete nursing package. She has Clare Ann's skills and Laura's kindness. She's lively, interested in everyone and everything. She's of medium build with brown hair and bright brown eyes. Her heels click rapidly as she walks. You can hear her coming a mile away. She thinks of herself as a partner to the patient, not an adversary. Ten minutes after she starts, I want her as my full-time nurse. It's love at first sight for me.

"Just let me know when you need to be turned again," she says. "You should be comfortable." Is she real?

Rikki warms to her immediately, telling her how we had enjoyed touring Ireland. "I'll be there next week," Kathleen says, describing her long-planned month's vacation. There go my dreams.

The three days with Kathleen are the happiest I've had since being sick. She tells me that I'm a good patient, not much trouble at all. Clare Ann should hear this.

When she leaves on her final day, she kisses me goodbye.

It's hard for me not to cry. I'm going to get her back, if it is at all possible. Rikki has already talked to her about working full time for me. Kathleen has made no promises but she has given Rikki her home phone number.

My stepmother has sent us a marvelous picture of my father in a straw hat. It captures his humor and kindness. It's large enough for me to see easily from my bed. It cheers me to look at it.

I did 790 cc's on my latest vital capacity test! When I can do 1,000 for a couple of weeks in a row they'll start weaning me from the respirator. Dr. Schick says that it shouldn't be long now. As soon as I can survive without a machine, it's on to rehab and goodbye forever, Clare Ann.

I can breathe without it for nearly five minutes at a time. Each breath takes a conscious effort. I also now have the reassurance of knowing that I can click my tongue for help.

Charlie is home on a vacation. He's overjoyed by all the progress I've made, how much I'm able to move. I do kind of a little jig in bed for him with my head and shoulders, making him laugh. He's spending most of his time looking for a summer job in graphic design. My condition no longer upsets him.

More visitors. Rikki's father comes for the first time. I can see he is shocked, but I know he'll adjust to seeing me like this. People do. Even Rikki's sister, Jinx, and her husband, Howard, who have been here again, are getting used to the machine and me. Howard is restoring a wood-bodied 1937 Ford station wagon. They hope to drive me to the rehab hospital in it. Maybe this time I won't need an ambulance. I'll ride in style instead.

Mornings I have a session in the chair (I'm up twenty miserable minutes at a time) and I watch television. If it's off,

I'm terribly bored and lonely. The best I can do are reruns of "The Love Boat." It's either that or a game show or soap operas. At least "The Love Boat" episodes have multiple plots. If you don't like one, ignore it and concentrate on another.

The ship cruises Mexico's Pacific coast. I'm always searching the port scenes for places we've been, but all they show are glimpses of stock shots. Even those are enough to get me daydreaming about Mexico and my father. It shouldn't be long now before we're there. I've started breathing on my own!

The Love Boat has docked and the news at noon is on. Rikki is late—probably trouble parking. That's a constant hassle. I hope that gets easier for her when I go to the rehab hospital. I'm anxious to see her. This morning has dragged.

Here she comes now. Oh, no, something is dreadfully wrong! Tears glisten on her cheeks. Her face is swollen, contorted and ugly from crying. She is clutching my hand. "Bob, darling," she says, "I have terrible news. Louise called this morning. Your father died last night…" I don't register the rest. I'm staggered, overwhelmed by monstrous grief and guilt. We loved each other so. We'll never be together again.

I'm sure he thought the optimistic reports about me were just tales they were telling to comfort an old man. He suffered too much grief. My mother died, Joan and Hanser and so many other friends – all dead. Now Bobby is dying too, he must have thought.

He was wrong. He should have waited. I'd have shown him that I'd beaten this thing and was myself again. If I needed it, I'd have bought a colorful Mexican cane like his. We'd have clowned with soft shoe routines. Now he's gone. My father is dead!

I cry silently. Rikki blots my tears with a tissue. The room seems eerily still, except for the sound of the respirator.

Suddenly its klaxon horn screams, startling us both. Rikki panics, racing out of the room to find a floor nurse. My tears have loosened a torrent of secretions.

The nurse is suctioning me too slowly. My fingers and toes tingle from lack of oxygen, but I no longer care. My father is dead! If I hadn't gotten sick, he'd still be living. I let him down, failed him, and now he's dead.

He died in a Cuernavaca hospital, Rikki is saying. He had been there several days, but Louise had kept the news from us. Many things had gone wrong with him at once. I wonder if he was frightened. I wonder if he knew what was happening. I'll bet the bastard doctors had their tubes in him too.

Louise is all alone. What am I going to do about her? She needs my help. I want to talk with her but that's impossible. I cannot talk to anyone. There's a funeral, financial matters. What a mess. Louise isn't organized. She drinks too much. She could go completely to pieces. I should be there. It's my job, my responsibility and I'm letting her down too. I've failed everyone. I'm useless, a fucking vegetable, that's what I am, and now I manage to kill my own father. They should have let me die!

"Your father had a wonderful life," Rikki sobs. "You made him so proud." My father is dead. I killed him!

"I'm very sorry about your father, Robert," Clare Ann sobs, embracing me, weeping. At first I don't comprehend what she's saying. Then I understand and a fresh flood of tears pours from me. It's true! My father is dead. Even Clare Ann knows. She kisses me, actually kisses me, on the lips.

I can't breathe! Jesus, I need to be suctioned now! She understands. She moves fast, jamming a catheter into my trach, sucking everything from me.

I'm numb. I don't want to go on. Why live? If there is a hereafter, I would be with my father. He'd welcome me with a wisecrack, a joke, an anecdote. There is nothing after death—nothing. I am never going to see my father again. That's the terrible reality.

Everything decays, wears out, wears down, dies. Nothing lasts. Even the Rocky Mountains will disappear. Everything you love is temporary. My father is dead!

"Do you want to skip the chair this afternoon?" Clare Ann asks in a whisper. Yes, I flash, confused by her kindness until I recall that her father died last year. For once, she knows how I feel.

Somehow this terrible afternoon is passing. Rikki is ready to leave. I'm terrified that something violent will happen to her. I want to protect her, keep her safe. I imagine someone on the filthy, dark streets waiting to attack her.

My panic is growing. I fear for Charlie. He's driving around Maryland in our car. Rikki won't remember to mail him the recall notice she just received. I see the brakes locking, Charlie fighting the wheel, the car tumbling down an embankment. I have no control over anything!

I'm alone. Clare Ann is in the nurses' lounge with Laura, giving her the nightly report about me. The network news is on. How can there be news today? Only one event in the last twenty-four hours has any meaning.

"I was sorry to hear about your father, Robert," Laura says. Her words bring back all the pain of the afternoon. More tears, fresh eruptions of secretions.

Laura's parents have been dead for years. She doesn't seem to miss them. She never even mentions them. I'm not like her. I will miss my father for the rest of my life. A day won't pass without me remembering him. If I read a fine book, hear a funny story, or see a good ball game, I'll think of how he would have enjoyed it.

Time passes painfully. Each day brings more tears.

Going on is so hard. I don't want to see anyone. I'm afraid of bursting into tears if they should mention my father. I'm inconsolable. I cry all the time.

In the week since he died, Rikki has been trying to get *The New York Times* to publish his obituary. If I were well, it would have been in the paper by now, on the wires too. My father wanted no monument, not even a tombstone, but he expected an obituary in the *Times*. I can't even do this for him.

The chances they'll publish the obituary now are slim. It's becoming old news. I make myself wait for Rikki every day to learn if it's in the paper. I could ask Clare Ann to look in her copy, but I don't want her to know I even expect to see it. When I spot her paper sitting on the windowsill this morning, I can no longer control myself.

P-A-P-E-R, I spell. She's amazed. I haven't wanted to read anything because I can't hold a paper or a book or magazine and I can't turn pages.

"What part?" she asks.

O-B-I-T-U-A-R-I-E-S.

She finds the page. "Is this what you want?" she asks softly, her finger pointing to a one-column, two-line headline. She props the paper on a table in front of my stretcher-chair. I squint to read:

"Charles Samuels, 79;

"Journalist, Biographer"

G-L-A-S-S-E-S. I need my bifocals. I can't see small print without them. Rikki brought them in weeks ago in case I changed my mind about reading. Clare Ann finds the glasses and puts them on me, turning the grey fuzz into clear words.

"Charles Samuels, the journalist and biographer of Clark Gable, Tex Rickard and other celebrities died April 27 in Cuernavaca, Mexico, where he had lived in retirement the last several years. He was 79 years-old," I read dry-eyed.

It's a decent obituary. It gives him credit for most of the books he wrote and, inexplicably, one about Jackie Gleason he didn't write. It also mentions that he had worked with Ben Hecht and Billy Rose.

I ask to see the front page when I'm done. I'm surprised at the number of stories it has but I only glance at the headlines. All I can concentrate on now is getting back to bed. Nothing else matters. I signal Clare Ann. "Read the paper," she says. She wants me up longer, always longer. My eyes tear with anger.

Dr. Ramsbotham has put me through another incredibly painful set of EMG tests. "I expect you will make an ambulatory recovery, but you will probably walk with crutches or canes. We'll have to see," he tells us after studying the results. Will I need canes and crutches for the rest of my life? He doesn't say and I'm afraid to ask.

"If you work hard, you'll make a full recovery," Clare Ann argues passionately when he leaves. "He doesn't know what will happen." Neither do you, I think, but I want to believe her.

Stanley Spiegel, our friend who is a psychologist, has warned all along that I will probably have terrible nightmares. That's not happened, but recently I've been having disturbing dreams.

Everything is vivid and real in them. I feel the slope of the hill as I walk Ruffy, my fingers against the typewriter keys as I write, and the smoothness of Rikki's skin as I hold her in the night. In my dreams I am innocent. I know nothing of this illness and hospitals. Then I wake to reality. I am in a hospital, on a respirator and there's one more day to face with Clare Ann.

I weep in bitter disappointment. Stanley was wrong. My

dreams are only dreams. My life is the nightmare. My father is dead. Laura tries to console me. She blots my tears and suctions me.

I've developed a strange new habit of biting the air. For some reason, it infuriates Clare Ann. She's always ordering me not to do it. I tell her it's my hobby, and that it's less harmful than her hobby, smoking. She's not amused.

Lindy, my physical therapist, comes every weekday afternoon. Her visits break the boring hospital routine. Clare Ann doesn't like her, doesn't think she pushes me hard enough, but I love her.

A Mrs. Haber, a friend of an old friend of ours, runs the hospital's occupational therapy department. She's a large, pleasant-looking woman who seems very sympathetic. It's too early for me to get occupational therapy, she tells us when she visits. She hopes I'll be in the program before she retires in six weeks.

Isn't there anything she can do to help me now, Clare Ann asks. The stretcher-chair limits what she can do, Mrs. Haber explains. If I were in a conventional wheelchair, she might be able to set it up so I could move my arms, maybe even turn the pages of a book.

That's all Clare Ann needs to hear. Now she's pestering the physical therapy department for a wheelchair. We must wait. There's a chronic shortage of wheelchairs as there is with so many things at this world-famous hospital. I'm excited. Unless the wheelchair has nails sticking through its seat, it is going to be more comfortable than the stretcher-chair. And moving my arms, turning pages—how?

In less than a week, Clare Ann has found a wheelchair. It has a high, reclining back. That's an essential feature. If they were to try to sit me upright, I'd topple forward like an unstrung puppet.

I stare at the wheelchair. How the hell are they going to get me in it? It won't be as easy as moving me to the stretcher-chair. That's terrifying, but comparatively simple. The stretcher-chair goes flat and they raise the bed until it is level with it. Even so, it takes three nurses, using a sheet, to slide me into it or back. I'm always frightened, although nothing bad has happened in all this time. How many nurses will it take now? The wheelchair reclines, but I don't think it goes flat, and it's so much lower than the bed. They can't make the bed go down that far.

Of course, none of these problems occurs to Rikki. She sees the wheelchair as the next logical step toward my complete recovery. She's happy. "Are you looking forward to trying it?" she wants to know. Yes, I flash. But how, I wonder.

"Are you ready for your new wheelchair, Robert?" Clare Ann asks the next morning. I rapidly shift my eyes to the right. Let's go! She wheels in a decrepit-looking steel contraption which has chains dangling from an arm. Someone repainted it long ago with the same cheerless grey paint they use on much of the equipment.

"Robert, this is a Hoyer lift," Clare Ann says, without further explanation. She has another nurse helping her. They roll me one way, then the other on the bed, slipping a cloth under me. Now what, I wonder.

Clare Ann moves the Hoyer lift closer to the bed and lowers the arm. One of its swinging chains grazes my face. Watch it, I silently scream. They're hooking the chains to grommets in the cloth. Clare Ann is pumping the handle of the Hoyer lift. It has the same sound as a car jack and produces the same result. I'm rising! Oh, God, I'm in the air, legs dangling from this sling. I feel like cargo that longshoremen are unloading. Work on banana boat all night long!

Don't drop me! Please, don't drop me! I'm shifting my eyes back and forth to tell them how scared I am. If something slips and I crash to the floor, it will shatter my bones.

They've swung me over the wheelchair. Clare Ann is opening a small valve at the top of the machine to release some air. I'm slowly descending. She's trying to guide me. "Oh, Jesus!" she moans. I'm missing the chair! She's pumping frantically but not much happens until she remembers to close the valve. I'm back up high, very high, swinging slowly in the air.

"You scared, Robert?" she asks, laughing partially in relief. I must look strange up here. Yes, I flash. Damn right I'm scared. "Don't worry. We ain't gonna drop you." I'm not reassured. "Let's try again," she says.

Once more I slowly descend. "He's right over it," the other nurse reports as I close on the target.

"I see that," Clare Ann snaps, but I'm missing it again! The front edge of the seat is rubbing my back. I'm going to hit the floor!

"Jesus, Mary and Holy St. Joseph!" cries Clare Ann as my backside touches the floor. She's pumping furiously. I'm going up. Here comes another bunch of bananas out of the hold. Daylight come and I wanna go home.

Clare Ann's no quitter. We're going to try again. She's jerkily lowering me. I'm in terror, palms sweating. My ass is over the target once more. Bombs away! No, no, hold it! Clare Ann has an idea. She tells the other nurse to pull back on the sling as I go down. Okay, everything set.

Jesus, she's pulling back too much. I feel as if I'm going to pitch head first onto the floor. "Pull it back more!" Clare Ann shouts. She's definitely trying to kill me! She's out of her goddamn mind!

That did it—I'm in the wheelchair. The eagle has landed! I'm slumping alarmingly to my right, as if shot. Clare Ann quickly stuffs pillows around me, propping me up. She puts my arms on the armrests and my feet on the footrests. The chair is raked back, sort of like a beach chair.

"You comfortable, Robert?" she asks sarcastically. Yes, I flash. I am. Jesus, I am! I'm astonished by my answer. So is she. If this chair is comfortable, my life will be much easier. We won't be continually fighting. I'll' spend a lot of time here.

Oh, oh, my ass is starting to pain. Why was I so quick to tell her it was comfortable? I know there are pillows under me but it feels as though I'm sitting on cobblestones. Tell her that you're hurting before she leaves. No, no, no! I won't! I won't grovel and ask her to put me back in bed. I won't tell her. She'll only sneer. Oh, God, this is terrible!

She's suctioned me and straightened the room. "The Love Boat" theme is on, signaling her coffee break. I'll be trapped in this chair! I have no self-control. I'm flashing. I hate myself for giving in. I have no resolve. I am weak, no good. Get me out of this fucking chair!

"I thought you liked your new chair," she says, full of scorn. I thought I did too. "You want me to get you back to bed?" I stare, not answering. From her tone I know if I say yes, she'll say no. There is no way to win with this bitch.

"No answer, Robert?" she sighs loudly. "Well, then, if it's all right with you, I'm taking my break." No, I flash, yielding again to the pain.

"No?" she asks, raising her eyebrows in exaggerated amazement. No, I flash furiously. "I suppose that means you want me to postpone my break for your comfort?" Yes, yes, yes! Maybe she will—maybe she'll realize just how desperate I am.

"I'm sorry but I don't think you've given the chair a

chance. You have to try harder," she says, going out the door.

I gaze up at the television. "The Love Boat" is Mexico-bound as usual. Concentrate on that. The cruise stirs up memories of my father. Many times each day I lapse into deep depressions about him. When Rikki is here, I often cry unexpectedly.

If I cry now and need suctioning, Clare Ann will be furious. She'll say I'm crying because I'm in the chair. Think about something else. Here's a scene by the ship's swimming pool. How come they never show a sexy girl in a revealing bikini? I can't think about this. GET ME OUT OF THIS WHEELCHAIR NOW!

I'm clicking my tongue. I don't care if she comes in here and has a fucking fit. I'm suffering. Let her get off her ass. She's supposed to help me! That's her job.

"Something wrong, Robert?" Yes, I flash. "Let me guess—you want to go back to bed?" Yes. You're a genius. "Well Robert, you must have made a mistake. You've only been up ten minutes. You have another ten minutes to go."

She lied! She's been gone more than ten minutes. The love boat is docking. All the dumb little plots have been neatly resolved. The credits are rolling. I know I've been up more than a half-hour. She put me in this chair before the show started. FUCKING BITCH LIAR!

She has to come soon. She can't go to lunch until she gets me into bed and feeds me. She never misses lunch. Oh, God, another program is starting. Maybe something happened to her. Maybe I've been forgotten. I'm clicking now. Someone has to hear; someone has to come!

"I see you're still alive," she says, sauntering into the room, as though she's not late.

The same nurse is helping her. They've hooked the

chains to the sling. Clare Ann pumps the handle. Each stroke lifts me a little higher, bringing relief.

~

It's my third session in the chair. Mrs. Haber is here with tools and equipment. She quickly attaches two L-shaped metal rods to the back of the chair and hangs leather slings from them. Then she puts my arms in the slings. I feel like a puppet.

"Try moving your arms," she says. I try and much to my amazement my arms swing free. All the power is coming from my shoulders and none from my arms, but still my arms are in motion and I'm in control. I'm elated.

"That's not good," Mrs. Haber says, noticing my hands limply dangling. She puts leather wrist supports on me. Mrs. Haber knows her stuff. "I'll be back in a while to see how you're doing," she promises.

"Swing your arms, Robert," Clare Ann says each time she brings another nurse to the room. She's showing me off like a proud mother, but I know her joy won't last. She'll soon be angry because I'm going to ask her to put my arms down. I've had them up only a few minutes and the slings feel as if they're cutting into my flesh. It's depressing. Everything I try is painful.

I flash at Clare Ann, complaining about my arms. "You want to go back to bed now?" she asks, pretending to be incredulous. No, I answer, but of course I want that too. I just don't dare tell her. Instead, I stare at my arms. "You want them down?" Yes.

No chance of that happening. "You just got them up," she says, shutting off the discussion.

I'm clicking in protest. It feels as if the slings are rubbing my arms raw. "You don't want to get better, do you Robert?" Oh, God, she's starting that again. "Most people in your position would be happy just to move their arms, but not you. All you care about is your own comfort."

"How's he doing?" asks Mrs. Haber, interrupting as Clare Ann is hitting her stride.

"Robert's not happy," Clare Ann tells her with exaggerated sympathy. "He says his arms hurt. He wants them down."

"Well, let's see," says Mrs. Haber, slipping my arms from the slings. "Oh, my, look at this. These straps are hurting him. See how they cut into him. It must be very painful," she adds. I want to cheer.

"Just a little redness," Clare Ann shrugs.

"You may call that a little redness," Mrs. Haber replies angrily, "but if his arms were up much longer it could have caused a skin breakdown."

Clare Ann stares in speechless amazement. No one ever openly contradicts her. "Excuse me," she finally manages, walking out. I love it! I love it!

"I guess you don't care for your nurse much, do you?" Mrs. Haber asks when we're alone. No, I flash. "Well, I don't blame you," she says. Please tell me what to do. Tell me how to get rid of her. I plead with my eyes but she says nothing more. She's padding the splints and wrist supports with adhesive-backed sponge rubber.

"You mentioned about arranging it so the patient can read?" a stony-faced Clare Ann asks, returning to the room as Mrs. Haber repositions my arms. Clare Ann, still stung by Mrs. Haber's anger, is trying to show her up. She doesn't believe it will be possible for me to turn pages on my own. Nor do I.

"We'll give it a try," says Mrs. Haber, taping a cheap, wire bookstand to my hospital table and sliding an occupational therapy textbook into it.

"Now, just how does he turn pages?" asks Clare Ann, hoping Mrs. Haber will look like a fool.

"I'm getting to that." Mrs. Haber replies coolly. She takes an ordinary yellow pencil and pushes the point end into a pocket on my right wrist support. Then she sticks some putty on the eraser end of the pencil. Now she grabs my arm and guides it so the putty catches the page and carries it to the other side of the book holder. It's a complicated maneuver. "You try it," she tells me.

I want it to work. I want her to show up Clare Ann. I try repeatedly, but I can't even touch the page with the pencil. I don't have the strength or the coordination. "Don't worry," Mrs. Haber says. "You'll soon be able to manage it." Clare Ann looks smug. I'm sure she's glad I failed.

~

The filth on the windows of my room bothers Laura. She's brought her own Windex to wash away what is probably years of dirt. I make a feeble joke to her about having a nurse who does everything including windows, but I'm touched that she cares this much about me.

When Clare Ann finds out, she can't get over it. "The man is on a respirator, and that one worries about his windows," I hear her telling a floor nurse. Her new name for Laura is "Window Nurse." It's a joke, a joke with a bite.

If I am able to read, I should read, Clare Ann figures, even if it means she has to turn the pages for me. She flags down a volunteer who is pushing a book cart. The woman's forced cheerfulness turns to open-mouth horror when she sees me. I guess there aren't many patients on respirators who are interested in literature.

Clare Ann has little patience for do-gooders. "Is something the matter?" she inquires.

"What's wrong with him?" the woman asks in a trembling voice.

"He's sick, lady," Clare Ann tells her. "This here's a hospital. There are a lot of sick folks here." She flips though the books on the woman's cart until she finds a current Updike novel. It is something I would have chosen for myself. I suspect few nurses would even have heard of John Updike.

She opens the book to the first page. I stare at the type. Christ, what's happened to my eyes? I can't read the print! Too small, I spell. Did I ruin my eyes when I wasn't able to close them? If I go blind, I'll want to die!

"You probably need new glasses," Clare Ann says, guessing my fears. Maybe that's it. "They have large print books on the cart, Robert. You could read those."

The only one that appeals to me is one I'd read years ago, John F. Kennedy's *Profiles in Courage*. Before I have a chance to start it again, Rikki's here. She's thrilled to see me with a book, but now all I want is to get back to bed. I've been up more than twenty minutes, and I could scream with pain. Clare Ann gives in to me without an argument. It's lunchtime and she wants to go out.

"I'm so happy that you're reading," Rikki says excitedly when she's let back into the room. I'm lying comfortably on my side, pillows behind my back to hold me in place. "You're the old Bob, getting back to normal." I wish it were true. "This must be the first you've read since you got sick."

No, I remind her. "O-B-I-T," I start to spell but there is no need to go on. The tears are flowing freely again.

I should see a psychiatrist about my depression, Clare Ann says. She's asked Dr. Ramsbotham to recommend one. Rikki is insisting I see one only if I want to.

How could a psychiatrist help me? I can't talk, for Christ's sake! I'm not even able to tell Rikki how I feel. I can't spell out for a stranger what my father meant to me.

No, I tell Rikki, no psychiatrist. My answer does not make Clare Ann happy.

I have mixed feelings about shrinks. I once met an overbearing woman at a party who was in therapy and insisted everyone else should be too. If I had a problem, I would certainly consider it, I told her.

"But aren't you curious about the way your mind works?" she demanded.

"Sure, I'm curious. I'm curious about my rear end too," I replied, "but I wouldn't go to a proctologist just to have him check it out and tell me about it."

Getting me to see a psychiatrist has become Clare Ann's new cause. She has Laura, Dr. Ramsbotham and Dr. Schick all working on me. I half expect my pal Shaun, the respiratory technician, to ask me why I won't see a shrink.

"There's nothing to be ashamed of, Robert," Laura assures me. I'm not ashamed. I think it's remarkable that I've kept my sanity so far. Maybe a shrink should study me to learn how I've done it.

"Clare Ann spoke to me again about getting you to see the psychiatrist," Rikki says. Clare Ann is at lunch. She just spent a half-hour telling me that I should stop biting the air and that I won't get better unless I work harder. By working harder she means sitting in the chair longer. She blames me for my slow recovery. My problem isn't mental, I tell Rikki, it is Clare Ann. She's horrible to me. A psychiatrist can't help.

"I don't know what to do," Rikki says, starting to cry. Suddenly, I remember Kathleen Cunningham, that Irish nurse I'd liked so much. She must be back from Ireland by now. Call her tonight, I tell Rikki, and ask her to work for us. The possibility of that happening is so exhilarating that it lifts my spirits and makes the afternoon fly.

Oh, Jesus, nothing works out. As soon as we're alone the next day Rikki tells me Kathleen would love to take my case. but she's afraid other nurses will accuse her of patient stealing. "I explained it's us who want to get rid of Clare Ann and that it has nothing with her. She still said no. I begged but it didn't do any good. Kathleen really likes you," Rikki adds. "She told me to call her if Clare Ann takes some time off or leaves. I'm so sorry, darling."

You tried. It's not your fault, I tell her. Is there no way to rid ourselves of the bitch? Can't she be hit by a truck or something?

If there is a God, he has a twisted sense of humor. A truck plowed into the passenger side of Clare Ann's car when she went to move it at lunchtime. The car is demolished, but Clare Ann escaped without a scratch.

I didn't want her killed or even badly hurt—a broken arm or a sprained ankle would do. I was just hoping for something serious enough to get her off my case and clear the way for Kathleen.

I want to see a shrink. I've changed my mind. My hope is that when he hears about Clare Ann, he'll insist we get rid of her to save my sanity. She's the sick one. He ought to commit her!

Dr. Richard Clark, my psychiatrist, is very nervous on his first visit. H-E-L-L-O, I spell to open my analysis. He's better at understanding me than Dr. Ramsbotham, but it's going to take forever to tell him anything complicated or abstract.

I ask if he'd mind if Rikki stayed on as a translator. Not at all, he says gratefully.

Rikki gets right to the point, telling him how trapped we are by Clare Ann. L-E-C-T-U-R-E-S, I remind her. "That's right," she says. "She lectures Bob all the time."

"How do you feel when she lectures you?" he asks. How do you think I feel, I'd like to reply, but I'm too polite. H-U-M-I-L-I-A-T-E-D.

"Why do you suppose she treats him like this?"

"I think she enjoys having total power over people," Rikki tells him. "She asked to take care of Bob. She wants patients who are completely dependent on her. She specializes in Guillain-Barré cases."

It's not that simple, I want to say. If all she wants is control, why doesn't she specialize in coma patients? They're perfect, she's told me many times, because they're completely undemanding, but I know she doesn't want them.

It's not only control she wants, I suddenly realize. She nurses Guillain-Barré victims because they win her lavish praise since they usually recover quickly and completely. She's angry with me because I'm failing her by not getting better faster. She may even think they'll blame her if things drag on. She sure as hell doesn't want that to happen to her, the hospital's best nurse.

She's sure she's done everything a nurse could possibly do to help me. She's certain it's not her fault. It's my fault. I'm not trying hard enough. I have no discipline and I'm restless. Rikki shares the blame. She babies me. My friends have contributed too. She hates all of us for making her fail. It's not her fault!

"What have you done about getting someone to replace her?" asks Dr. Clark

We've tried, Rikki says, explaining the difficulties. T-R-A-P-P-E-D, I add unnecessarily

"Is that your main problem?" Dr. Clark asks me.

Y-E-S. I answer, not mentioning my father's death.

We've now had our third session with Dr. Clark. He's helped me understand Clare Ann, but he hasn't been able to do anything more about getting rid of her. I'm trying not to let that get me down. I've been making more progress toward recovery. I'm now able to mouth words clearly enough so people who can read lips understand what I'm saying. Clare Ann is good at this and Laura is fantastic, but Rikki finds it difficult. I still have to spell for her.

My breathing has improved enough to allow me to be off the machine for a half-hour at a time. This means I finally can leave the room and I'll soon be going upstairs to the physical therapy floor for treatments.

My first wheelchair trip out of my room is to the turret-like solarium at the end of the corridor. Its windows are open, bathing me in a soft, spring breeze. It's the first fresh air I've felt since early December. Rikki sits beside me. We look out at the Hudson River. Fluffy, white clouds dot a perfect blue sky. A tugboat pulls six empty barges upstream. My vision mists with tears. Don't cry, please don't cry, I plead with myself.

I mean nothing to the crew on the tug. My health, my life, is of no importance to them. I'm struck by the sudden painful knowledge of the world's indifference to my problems. Everyone I've seen for months has been totally concerned with my welfare. I'd forgotten there is a world that has nothing to do with me. I've been taken care of like a baby and, like an infant, I'm shocked to learn the universe doesn't revolve around me.

Every experience is new. It's even a novelty to get in an elevator for the quick ride upstairs to the therapy floor. Clare Ann says therapy will speed up my recovery. Before we leave the room she lectures me about my habit of biting the air.

It embarrasses her. I'm unaware of it when I do it but it is strangely satisfying.

On the therapy floor Clare Ann pushes me through a corridor and into a large, gym-like room alive with people, commotion and rock music. A woman in a wheelchair is pulling on ropes connected to weights. A man in running shorts is balancing between parallel bars on a pipe-like artificial leg. Therapists are working with patients on raised mats.

This place is filled with cripples! What am I doing here? I'm not like them. I will recover. How dare they send me here! I'm fighting back the tears. I don't want to be a part of this.

Rosemary Schneider, my new physical therapist, doesn't give me time to brood. She radiates overwhelming energy and enthusiasm. She knows I have Guillain-Barré and that means she knows I'm going to get better, not like the others. I don't want her to see me looking depressed.

Rosemary will work with me in the wheelchair this time but soon I'll be on one of the mats. She moves my arms and legs back and forth in the now familiar range-of-motion exercises. "Don't let him goof off," Clare Ann tells her, enraging me.

My first session is quickly over. Clare Ann is pushing me back to the elevator. "Robert, here's a mirror," she says. "Look how good you look."

At first I see only Clare Ann standing behind someone in a wheelchair. I don't recognize myself. Then I look more carefully. Am I that refugee from Buchenwald, that ghastly creature in the hospital gown? No! As I start to tell her it's not me, I notice the refugee is moving his lips. God, it is me!

"Don't you look terrific?" she asks, pointing. She's completely sincere. She really does think I look good. But I see a man who seems close to death; his chest is frail, his eyes deeply sunken. That's not the me I know. I'm healthy and robust. I try to change my blank expression to a frown, but my face remains frozen. I'm in turmoil, but I stare back at myself blandly. I can't change my expression. My own face is a mask.

I have a newly realized appreciation for my hospital room. It is my refuge, a place without shocks or surprises. Here people accept me, tell me how well I'm doing. I see no other patients, no pathetic cripples, no mirrors.

When Laura asks how my first session went, I say "fine" and change the subject. I want to forget about the rehab floor. In fact, I want to quit going, but I can't imagine Clare Ann or the doctors permitting that.

Each time I see the other patients I'm shocked by their condition but they hardly give me a second glance. It's as though they accept me as one of them. They don't know that I will make a full recovery.

For over a week now, I've been coming up to the therapy room for half-hour sessions. I'm ready to work on a mat, Rosemary says. I've been studying the mats, knowing this was coming, and I don't see how I'll ever get on one. They seem identical to gym mats except they're up on large, knee-high tables. They could move me with a Hoyer lift, but I haven't seen one on this floor. How? I ask, mouthing the word.

She'll stand-pivot me, Rosemary says, explaining it involves her lifting and swinging me onto the mat. To start, she puts my arms around her neck, but they immediately flop off. She has Clare Ann hold them in place.

"Don't be scared," Rosemary says, crouching in front of me. "We do this all the time. One, two," she begins, grasping me around the waist and rocking me back and forth in my wheelchair. My head rests on her shoulder. It's like dancing. I smell her clean, frizzy hair. On three, she yanks me out of my chair by the waist of my pajama pants and, in one terrifying maneuver, she swings me so I'm sitting on the side of the mat.

"Very good, Robert," says Clare Ann, as if I'd done it on my own.

Only Rosemary's strong arms keep me from crumbling to the floor. "Now I'm going to put you on your back," she says, pivoting me around and slowly lowering me. The mat is shockingly hard, not like the gym mats I remember from school, and all at once I'm choking. I can't breathe!

Rosemary runs for a portable suctioning machine. My breath comes in weak gasps, blocked by the mucus that clogs my trach, but I'm not the least bit frightened. This is routine. I always need suctioning when I lie down. I'm confident Clare Ann will soon have me breathing freely again.

The suctioning machine sounds a little strange, and the familiar pull isn't there as Clare Ann pushes the catheter into my trach. "Jesus, Mary and Holy St. Joseph," she explodes, "one of the hoses is missing!"

"I'll get another machine," says Rosemary, racing off. I sense everyone in the room is watching us. The only sound is Simon and Garfunkel on the radio, singing about a bridge over troubled water. It's scoring too corny for a movie. My fingers tingle from lack of oxygen.

"You ain't gonna die, Robert," Clare Ann says caustically. I'm not worried about that. She's sure not going to let me die and take the blame. What I am worried about is brain damage from the lack of oxygen. What's taking so long? Where's Rosemary?

Clare Ann should have checked the suctioning machine before I lay down. I'll bet she didn't think of it. Miss Perfect fucked up. I know she has an ambu bag. She brings one each time I leave the room in case something like this happens. She's too stubborn to use it now. She won't admit this is an emergency! She's like a lost motorist who refuses to ask for directions. Christ, use the damn bag!

Everything is moving in slow motion except the black spots dancing crazily before my eyes. Rosemary has found another suctioning machine. Clare Ann is ripping the crinkly sterile bread-stick paper off a fresh catheter. She shoves the catheter into my trach. It's sucking me clear. Clare Ann pauses before shoving it in a second time. She thinks she's giving me a chance to catch my breath but it's too late—I'm blacking out.

Suddenly, she's jamming the ambu bag onto my neck, squeezing it, forcing fat blasts of air through my trach and into my lungs. I'm feeling better already, but God, I wonder if I get a little dumber each time this happens.

"That's enough for today," says Rosemary, sitting me back up on the side of the mat, her face glistening with sweat. I'm glad to be off my back.

"There's no need to stop the session," Clare Ann protests. "He just needed a little suctioning. He's okay now."

"Do you want to continue?" Rosemary asks me. I don't want to be on that hard mat again, but if I say that Clare Ann will say I'm a quitter. I have Vince Lombardi for a nurse!

"We'd better stop for today," Rosemary decides before I'm forced to answer.

Another stand-pivot rockets me back into the wheelchair. Clare Ann quickly collects my chart and the ambu bag and starts pushing through the therapy room to the corridor. The other therapists and patients are still frozen, staring at me in shock.

Marge Bauer, a neighbor from home who works part time for a medical researcher here, occasionally stops in. We were never good friends. I'm sure it wouldn't occur to her to visit if it weren't so convenient. Even so, I've gotten to enjoy seeing her. She manages to come when no one else is here, and she talks interestingly about people and places I know.

Marge is different today, less tired, and more anxious to see me. "I'm going to tell you something I haven't told anyone else," she begins conspiratorially, making me very uneasy because I don't feel close enough to her to hear her secrets.

"I have wonderful news. My doctor just told me that Bill and I are going to have twins. I haven't been able to reach Bill yet and no one else even knows I'm pregnant." I swing my eyes back and forth, trying to tell her I share her excitement.

"I can confide in you because you can't repeat it," she says with a sly smile. But I can. I feel like a character in a farce who everyone mistakenly assumes is a eunuch. My potential for mischief is limitless.

Clare Ann's learned that Carla, a giggly Asian floor nurse, reads palms, so she's dragged her in to read mine. Clare Ann has more faith in this stuff than she has in medicine. Carla seems a little simple but very sweet. Her brow furrows as she studies my hand. I'm a total skeptic, but please don't tell me if it's bad news.

Carla breaks into a wide grin. "Your future very good!" she says. My lifeline is very long but it has a little zigzag in the middle. I'm living that part now, she explains. Some zigzag! Once I'm through it, it's clear sailing to the end, and that end is a long way off, she promises. Clare Ann is beaming with joy. This means more to her than anything a doctor could say.

Near the last part of each shift, Clare Ann has been getting me up and letting Laura put me back to bed. She thinks she's increasing the amount of time I'm in the wheelchair, but she's mistaken. I'm so miserably uncomfortable that as soon as I see Laura, I start begging her to get me out of the chair.

Laura is a sweetheart. She always puts me to bed as soon as she can find someone to help her. I love the relief I feel as the Hoyer lift slowly pulls me up off the chair. If I thought they'd listen to me, I'd ask the nurses to pump the handle very slowly just to stretch out my pleasure. I'm a Hoyer lift junkie.

"What's this?" demands Clare Ann, returning unexpectedly. "Is there something wrong with the patient?" She stares at me in mock amazement as I hang in my sling. She knows damn well there's nothing wrong.

"Everything's okay," Laura says. "He was uncomfortable, so I'm putting him back to bed."

"You're putting him back to bed because he's uncomfortable? You can't listen to him. He's always uncomfortable. He never wants to be up."

Clare Ann will never understand the pain I have when I'm sitting up. The first fifteen minutes or so are fine, but then I start to hurt, first my backside, then the rest of me. Gravity grinds me down, crushes me because I have no muscles to pad my bones. I wish it was different; I wish there was no pain.

I'm now reading by myself, but it's not easy. It takes me many attempts to turn a single page. If one slips out of the bookstand, I have to call Clare Ann for help. She claims I do it deliberately just to have an excuse to click my tongue to get her back to the room. Sometimes that's just what I'm doing. I hope once she's here, she'll put me back to bed. She seldom does.

If I could stand the pain, I'd spend all my time in the chair reading. I must be up more than she admits because I've finished *Profiles in Courage,* and I'm into the large-type version of some early Steinbeck. I haven't read him in years, but I'm finding I still love his stuff.

"You have to stay up at least fifteen-minutes longer," Laura says the next night without explanation or apology. No amount of silent pleading or whining does any good. Clare Ann has spoken.

Laura wants me to visit the solarium with her. No, I don't want to go that far from the bed. She's never seen me any place but this room, she argues. Besides, I might enjoy the change of scene. Okay, I tell her. It's hard to say no to her because she has so often said yes to me.

Soon she's happily pushing me down the hall. When we get there, I'm immediately glad we've come. There's a spectacular sunset, the first I've seen since I've been in a hospital. The massive apartment buildings topping the New Jersey palisade cliffs across the Hudson stand silhouetted in the fading purple light.

As a boy living on Manhattan's west side, I had nearly the same view. I imagined the brown palisades were carved dark chocolate. In my mind they marked the abrupt end of the city and the beginning of the country. The illustrations in all my books confirmed that cities end suddenly, with tall buildings on one block and rolling pastures the next. The apartment towers that top the New Jersey cliffs today make New York seem like a city without end.

Palisades Amusement Park was one of the few interruptions in the cliff's natural ridgeline then. White lights traced the park's rides, giving upper Manhattan kids a nightly view of paradise every summer. At least once every year my parents, sister and I would heed the words of the park's bouncy radio commercial and "come on over." It was an inexpensive outing for my parents because the park's press agent, an old friend of my father's, sent them free passes.

The journey to New Jersey (a different state!) was an adventure. We took a ferry across the river. The bus ride up the cliff road was scary, totally unlike a usual bus ride on flat city streets. As we got close,

I'd stare up at the powdery white roller coaster.

Those days always seemed sunny and perfect. It's all gone now, demolished for apartments. Fate had the same ending for two New York ballparks, the Polo Grounds and Ebbetts Field—both happy places I loved as a kid.

Today the weather is warm enough for Clare Ann to take me outside. As long as she brings the ambu bag, there's no reason not to, she says. We wait for Rikki who gets giddy when she hears the plan. It's another step toward full recovery!

It has been so long since I've been outside that the prospect makes me feel like Rip Van Winkle waking from his long nap. Will I recognize anything? Will cars look different? Down we go in the elevator. People rush by in the lobby, normal people not giving me a glance. Rikki is so excited. She's introducing me to a cheerful Puerto Rican security guard who tells me what a wonderful girl I married. I can't argue with that.

He grandly holds the door open for us, and in walks Sally Savage, an old friend. She was just coming for a visit. Lucky she's spotted us. Sure, she'd love to come along.

The street is not at all familiar. It's quieter than I imagined. On the other side is a handsome, modern hospital building that I didn't expect. Clare Ann has parked me sideways on a sloping sidewalk. She sits on a low wall near Rikki and Sally. Both Rikki and Clare Ann have lit cigarettes, the first I've seen anyone smoke since I've been sick. It bothers me a little that Rikki's gone back to it, but I'm sure I would have done the same if I'd had her pressures.

I marvel at the pedestrians and at what traffic there is. It's all so mundane to everyone but me. It's like the first time I saw a London cop. "That's a real London bobby, a real London bobby," I kept idiotically repeating to myself. I feel like that now.

Sally Savage is a dear, but she has no way of understanding how much this first trip outside means to me. She's chatting on to Rikki about her own life and problems. God, I hope they don't notice that my eyes are filled with tears. I'm overcome by feelings of loss. The world has gone on without me.

Because I'm on a slant, the left side of my buttocks is being ground into the wheelchair. I suddenly want to go in. I want to get back to bed. I'm twisting my head side-to-side for attention. "What's wrong, Robert?" Clare Ann asks.

Bed, I mouth. Pain!

"Stay out a little longer," she urges pleasantly. "Enjoy yourself."

"Isn't this wonderful, darling?" Rikki says. "It's so nice to be outside with you."

"It's a marvelous day," adds Sally.

I want to scream, cry, and beat my fists. No one can imagine the pain.

~

We haven't been out again for several days but Clare Ann is surprising me this morning by taking me across the street to a small art gallery where Rikki has several pieces of calligraphy art. We'll also see a canvas of a nude named "Clare Ann." The male nurse who painted it titled it that as a joke. Clare Ann swears she didn't pose for it. That's a relief.

It is bright and breezy, not as warm as last week but nice enough. The steep pitch of the sidewalk near the entrance hadn't been a problem then. It tilts down toward the building's u-shaped driveway to allow rain to run off. The driveway climbs a short but steep hill to the front door.

My wheelchair is heavy, making it difficult to control. Clare Ann's as strong as she can be, but she's just not tall enough to have any leverage. She's struggling to get me down the sidewalk and I'm terrified. The chair could easily slip away and crash over the high curb. I'm completely defenseless. I can't even raise a hand from my lapboard to protect myself.

Thank God we're at the end of the driveway, on level sidewalk. Oh, Jesus, we have to cross the street. She's started me down an insanely steep curb cut. I feel as though I'm going to pitch forward out of the chair. Now she's pushing me across the street, unaware of my fears.

Oh, Christ, there's no cut on this side. She's grunting, tilting the chair back to get me up the high curb, but she's not strong enough. What do you know, there's Shaun, the respiratory therapist. He's rushing to help.

Shaun's gotten me safely on the sidewalk, but he's left us. The surface here is level and smooth. Hope the gallery isn't far. It's supposed to be across the street from the hospital but that could mean anything now.

"Here we are, Robert," Clare Ann says, turning in at a storefront unexpectedly. Now she's having problems with the glass door. She has to hold it while pulling me through, no easy trick. My chair bangs against the frame, but finally we're inside. I never knew pushing a wheelchair was so difficult.

It's much darker here than anywhere in the hospital. Only the paintings are well lit. There's Rikki's stuff. I always know her pictures. One is a drawing of a cat made from words about cats, and the other is a Monopoly board with local street names. "Those are very nice," Clare Ann says with surprise.

We've moved slowly around the small gallery to the "Clare Ann" painting. It sure isn't a portrait of her. The model is heavier and bustier. "It's very good, Robert, don't you think?" I nod in agreement. It's not the "Mona Lisa," but it's not bad. I can see that the title thrills Clare Ann. Mona Lisa couldn't have been happier.

"Don't you enjoy being away from the hospital?" she asks. Yes, I tell her but I'm gripped with worry over how she'll get me back. How will she manage that first curb? She doesn't even realize it's a problem.

When we reach it she just shoves the chair over the edge. The wheelchair rocks then lands violently, slamming me forward, my head crashing down on my lapboard. I feel like someone punched me in the mouth.

"You're okay, Robert. You're okay," she's saying even before she has a chance to see if I am. She is pulling me back up to a sitting position and straightening my glasses. They're badly askew. I'm too numb with fear to know if I've been hurt.

"They need a curb cut there," she notes needlessly as she stoops to retrieve the ambu bag. It had bounced into the gutter like a fumbled football.

The curb on the other side has the too-steep cut, but that's not a danger now because we're going up it. I'm breathing easy. She's handling the tough slope of the sidewalk better than I expected. We're going to make it. She's pulling at the door to the hospital with one hand and trying to hold onto my chair with the other. Oh, my God! The chair is getting away from her! I've spun completely around and I'm rolling toward the curb! My footrests are over the edge! I'm going to break my neck!

Suddenly, a white-jacketed young man is grabbing for the arm of my chair. He has it! He spins me back and pushes me up the walk and inside the building as Clare Ann holds the door. "Thanks," she says, as if he'd done us a minor favor. She should be groveling at his feet. He saved my life!

"No problem," he shrugs, walking off. Can't he see how careless she was? He should report her, turn her in, get her fired!

"Now that the weather is good, we'll be going out every day," Clare Ann promises, as cheerful as the first spring robin. Is she out of her fucking mind? I was within an inch of the edge. I never want to go outside again. My palms sweat with the memory. Two of my teeth are loose from hitting the lapboard.

~

"Can we go back outside this afternoon?" Rikki asks when she finds I missed seeing one of her paintings. No! No! I wouldn't go back if I'd missed a Van Gogh and they promised to give it to me as a present if I returned.

"Let's wait until tomorrow," says Clare Ann. I try to seem disappointed. If she learns I'm afraid, she'll be forcing me outside several times a day. I can't tell Rikki my fears. She might let it slip.

Good news! The weatherman on the six o'clock news is predicting heavy rain for tomorrow. That will keep us inside. Let it rain all summer. No farmer ever wished for rain more than I do now. They're only trying to save their crops; I'm trying to save my life.

There's no end to this. Laura wants to take me out soon too. My palms are sweating again. She'd be worse with the wheelchair than Clare Ann. She's more cautious, but she's not as strong.

I sleep poorly—nightmares of crashing off the curb. When I wake, it's pouring. Let it rain for a month! We'll visit the gallery some other time, I tell Rikki. We have the rest of the spring. Oh, Jesus, keep raining!

Not going out has been easier than I would have imagined. There's always an excuse, often supplied by Clare Ann. "I'd take you today but its too hot," she'll say. Or, "I'd take you out but we don't have the time." Maybe she's afraid too.

All I have to do to get Rikki to stay in is to remind her that we'll have to take Clare Ann with us. Laura's suggestions about going out for evening walks have proven empty. I think she's frightened to try it. The one time she suggested it, I said I'd rather visit the solarium. She looked relieved.

Mornings now I go to the rehabilitation floor for occupational therapy. My therapist, Rhoda Levin, a tall, thin blonde girl from Brooklyn, has no trouble reading my lips, so we converse easily.

Rhoda ranges my joints, from my shoulders to the tips of my fingers, bending them and flexing them in every possible direction, keeping them loose for the day I start moving them myself. Will I be able to play the piano? I joke.

"Oh," she asks with concern, "did you play the piano well?" Never played a note, I tell her, embarrassed that I fooled her, but she thinks I'm funny.

My physical therapist, Rosemary Schneider, is away this week so Arthur Zuckerman, her boss and the head physical therapist, has been working with me on the mats. He has some difficulty adjusting to my weakness, but he's extremely professional. He also has a good sense of humor.

Do you think I'll ever walk again? I ask, trying a joke similar to the one I made with Rhoda.

He looks grave. "No one can tell for sure," he answers. He doesn't find my question funny. He's acting as if there's doubt and he shouldn't build up any false hopes. Jesus, what if I don't walk! But no one else questions if I'll walk. He must not know about Guillain-Barré.

Charlie, home on spring break, has some great news. He's found a job as an assistant in a New York graphics arts studio. It's just what he's been looking for, and, what's more, he even has a place in the city to live for the summer.

Dr. Ramsbotham wants to give me another EMG to test the phrenic nerve in my neck. He says it will tell him why I've been so slow to resume breathing on my own. He doesn't have to tell me that sending jolts through needles in my neck will be very painful.

Rikki's angry. She thinks I've become a too willing guinea pig. "You can say no," she tells me.

I should take the test, be cooperative, Laura urges. Of course she'd tell me that. She'd want me to have a frontal lobotomy if some doctor recommended it.

"Most people go along with their doctor," Clare Ann says, relishing my dilemma. She knows my opinion of Dr. Ramsbotham and maybe even shares it. What do you think I should do? I ask. She claims not to care. "You should do what you think is best, Robert. You have a right to refuse, but I don't think you will. You don't have the guts."

Guts—it takes more guts to go through with the test. I'm only trying to do the right thing. I want to do what the doctors say and get better.

This is the day. I'm on a stretcher. Clare Ann pushes me into the elevator and up we ride, past the therapy floor, to the floor where they give the test. He has done all my previous EMG's in my room because I couldn't be away from the respirator.

The testing room is tiny, a cell. Clare Ann finds an attendant to help her slide me onto a hard table. The stretcher was uncomfortable but this is much worse. We wait. I hate it. I'm on my back, in pain, harsh florescent lights glaring in my eyes. I wish I were back in my room. I wish I'd said "no" to the test.

Finally, the door swings open and a doctor with a Van Dyke and a white coat ambles in. Dr. Ramsbotham, he says, is busy so he's going to test me. I want Dr. Ramsbotham. He may be a bumbler, but he's a gentle bumbler. I'm too polite to tell the Van Dyke to go away.

A younger, clean-shaven doctor joins the Van Dyke. He'll assist. They're sticking the small needles into my neck and chest, wiring me to the machine. I no longer exist for them as a person, if I ever did. They're discussing some hospital scandal, someone sleeping with someone, as though they're alone. Then the Van Dyke tells his assistant that Dr. Ramsbotham hates causing pain so he always finds someone else to give this test.

Now they're ready. They've turned off the overhead lights, not for my comfort but because the brightness makes it difficult for them to read the dials on their instruments.

The zaps begin, slowly and weakly at first, and then they pick up. The jolts are making the muscles in my neck jump and burn. I'm surprised I don't smell smoldering flesh. The pain is horrible. I'm weeping. If I could, I'd be howling.

"Hold on," the Van Dyke tells me impatiently. Hold on how, you stupid shit. My hands don't work, nothing works, and my father is dead! He'd kill you if he could see what you're doing to me.

My tears prime other secretions. Once again I'm choking, unable to breathe. The doctors are panicking, pushing open the door, calling Clare Ann who by now must be relaxing somewhere with coffee, a cigarette and *The New York Times*. I'm sure there's no suction machine on this floor, but I'm wrong. I hear the squeaky wheels of a portable machine someone found somewhere. Clare Ann has it and it works! Amazing!

They're back zapping, moving the needles to different places in my neck, testing various sections of the nerve, repeating their experiment, talking on about the scandal. I'm fighting to hold back the tears. Tears only slow things down. Finally, it's over.

"How was the test?" Rikki asks. Horrible, I tell her. "You didn't have to have it," she reminds me. Why don't you go to hell! I cry. Just go home and leave me alone! My rage baffles her.

"I'm sorry you found the test uncomfortable," Dr. Ramsbotham says, on his afternoon visit. I wasn't uncomfortable, I was in pain, I want to say.

What were the results? I ask, mouthing the words.

"Oh, dear, what is he saying?" he asks Clare Ann.

"Robert wants to know the results of the test," she tells him.

"Oh yes, quite. The test show that your breathing is continuing to slowly improve."

You didn't need a fucking EMG for that, you dumb bastard, I want to scream. You can measure my breathing just by looking at me. If you need scientific proof, look at my vital capacity test results.

Clare Ann is away for three days. As usual, she gave no advanced warning so Rikki was unable to get Kathleen Cunningham, the Irish nurse, as a substitute, but things have worked out. The registry sent Rosa, that good Filipina nurse who took care of me Super Bowl Sunday. She can't get over how much I've improved.

Dr. Schick is here listening to my chest. She's trying to detect movement in my diaphragm. "Not yet," she concludes. Her examination, she says, confirms the EMG test. It showed that my phrenic nerve, which I gather connects the diaphragm to the rest of the nervous system, remains short-circuited. The EMG can't predict when I will recover, she adds. Then why did they do it?

Isn't my diaphragm the muscle that moves my lungs?

I ask. Yes, she says. Well, if it isn't working, how do I breathe without it? I say, mouthing the words.

"Your rib muscles are doing the work, which is fine for now," she explains. "The long-term drawback is that rib muscles, unlike the diaphragm, can't function automatically. Each breath requires a conscious effort."

What happens if I fall asleep when I'm off the respirator? I mouthed. Could I die?

"It's possible," she says, as if she's discussing the likelihood of rain tomorrow. Holy shit!

Every morning after occupational therapy Clare Ann puts me back to bed, reattaches the respirator and leaves for lunch. Since Rikki comes in later now, I use the time to take a nap. But Clare Ann wants to change things. She plans to leave me off the respirator for the hour she's away. The idea is to have me breathe on my own, for longer periods. I beg her not to do it.

"Are you afraid you'll stop breathing if I'm not around?" she asks mockingly.

Yes, I tell her. When you were away, Dr. Schick told me my diaphragm isn't working. She said I could die if I fell asleep off the respirator because I have to make a conscious effort to breathe.

"That's nonsense," says Clare Ann. "Were you conscious of breathing while you've been telling me all this?" she asks. No, I admit.

"Do you think about breathing when you're in physical therapy?" No.

"Robert, your diaphragm is working," she assures me. "Relax, you ain't going to die if you fall asleep." She's putting her blue trench coat on over her reindeer sweater. "Someone will look in on you while I'm away," she says.

She's right—I don't think about breathing. But what does she really know? She's no doctor. She wasn't even aware x-rays are dangerous. I wish I could ask Dr. Schick to talk to Clare Ann about my breathing, but she's away on vacation. There's no point in asking Dr. Ramsbotham. He never has any answers. If I tried to spell it all out to Rikki, I'd have to start by explaining what the diaphragm is. I'll ask Laura. She'll know something.

Laura is appalled. She can't believe that Clare Ann would be irresponsible enough to leave me off the respirator when there's a chance of my falling asleep. "I'm sure Clare Ann wants you to stay awake while she's gone," she says hopefully.

Oh no, I mouth, she thinks it's fine if I sleep. But don't worry—I couldn't fall asleep if I tried. I'm too tense for that. I'll stay awake, I promise.

I can't keep that promise. I wake with a start the third lunch hour I'm off the respirator. I nodded off. Why didn't I die? How was I able to breathe? Doesn't Dr. Schick know anything?

Dr. Schick is back from her vacation at last. She's listening to my chest with her fancy, two-headed stereo stethoscope. Is my diaphragm working? I ask anxiously. "Not yet." Then how am I able to sleep without the respirator? I demand.

"You can't sleep for long without it," she says. But you said I could die. "You could," she answers as her beeper sounds and she runs off to some emergency.

"I don't care what she says," Clare Ann tells me as soon as we're alone, "your diaphragm is working. I'm with you twelve hours a day. I see how you breathe on your own for long periods. She doesn't."

I'm in the solarium with Rikki, hooked to a small, portable respirator that Dr. Schick wanted me to try. It seems to work fine. I've adjusted to it, forgotten it's breathing for me, and then suddenly it goes berserk. It's filling my lungs, not letting me exhale! Oh, God, my lungs will explode!

Rikki's frantic. She sees I'm terrified, but she doesn't understand why. I'm twisting my head violently, shaking the respirator hose free. Air blasts from my trach.

My heart's racing with fear. This time both my lungs may have ripped. "Should I put the hose back on you?" Rikki asks over the piercing squeal of the respirator's alarm. No. I can breathe on my own for several hours if I have to.

Are you okay?" Yes. "Do you need Clare Ann?" Yes.

Clare Ann checks my finger nails to see if they're turning blue from lack of oxygen. They're okay. She thinks I'm exaggerating what happened. "Let's try the machine again," she suggests. No, I tell her, no way.

The damn thing works perfectly when Dr. Schick comes. "Will you try it again?" she asks. No! She's using all her considerable charm, trying to sell me on it. I'm not charmed. She won't give up. She's describing the safety features. I'm unimpressed. What I think happened couldn't have happened, she says. It happened. She has to leave. Thank God she's taking the machine with her.

I've lost all faith in her. She is responsible for much that has gone wrong. In the beginning, she wouldn't let herself see that Pearl knew nothing about respirators. That almost killed me. She tore my lung by increasing the respirator settings. She ordered those crazy beds and caused me hours of misery. She wants me to try the portable respirator again, even though she doesn't know what's wrong with it.

She'll tell me anything. She said I'd be able to eat sooner if they removed my nose tube. It's obvious now she made that up to get me to agree to the stomach tube. She scared me unnecessarily about falling asleep off the respirator.

No one here seems to know what they're doing! I'm at one of the world's most famous hospitals and my nurse has more faith in palm readers than she does in the doctors and I can't blame her.

Weekends now I have many visitors.

Davis and Cynthia Crippen, a couple our age who are old friends, come frequently, and when their sons, Tom and Alex, are home from college they bring them along.

The Crippens are very verbal. Tom has literary ambitions; Alex is heading for a journalism career; Cynthia is a book indexer; and Davis has worked in publishing and public relations. When I spell, they're the most competitive at guessing what I mean. Each wants to be first. I feel like the hottest thing in new board games.

This Sunday afternoon Dick Howe, another friend of many years, is visiting us. He's scooting merrily around on an old-style wooden wheelchair that he found in the hall. He's obviously comfortable even though he's sitting on a cane seat. That would be screamingly painful for me. Jesus, I was able to sit on cane chairs. I've forgotten what's normal.

Why does it hurt so much when I sit, I finally ask Rosemary Schneider, my physical therapist. "You don't have any muscles in your butt," she explains. "That's what gives a normal person padding and allows them to shift their weight."

I try telling this to Clare Ann. "You should ignore the pain," she says.

"Robert, do you like soft shell crabs?" Clare Ann asks late one afternoon. I adore them, but how is she going to feed them to me? She can't shove them down my stomach tube. No, she's just bragging and tormenting me. She's on her way to a soft shell crab festival in lower Manhattan.

"Do you ever want to try eating?" she asks three days later. Yes. "What would you like?" Soft shell crabs, I mouth.

"What?" she asks again, not understanding my joke. Soft shell crabs, I repeat. "You'll have to wait until you're better for those," she says seriously. My menu choices for my first taste of food, are ice cream, Jell-O, or something pureed in a blender. I pick ice cream, which happens to be the last food I tasted at Nyack Hospital six months ago.

I thought she was talking about me eating sometime in the vague future, but here she is with a Dixie cup. She puts some vanilla on a wooden tongue depressor and slips it into my mouth. The cold sweetness is startling wonderful, but after three tiny bites I'm exhausted from swallowing. Still, it's progress! I'm recovering!

I'm eating a little more everyday now. After the ice cream, she has ordered pureed food. I don't like it. "It is the same as regular food. This is how it looks once it's in your stomach," she points out. That is precisely why it's revolting.

I do like the soft-boiled eggs and some of the other things she's ordering, but mostly eating has turned out to be a pain. She hates cutting everything up for me. She's always forcing me to eat more than I want. If I'm ever going to have the tube taken out of my stomach, I must be able to eat enough to stay alive, she harps. She loves having a reason to nag me.

I used to fantasize with Warren Jones, my best friend, boss, and lunchtime companion at Texaco, about how marvelous it would be if a doctor ordered us to eat more. Well, it came true for me and it's not marvelous.

I don't remind Warren of that when I finally let him visit. He is shocked at seeing me as everyone is but I think he enjoys himself. He told me the latest office jokes and brought me copies of *The Texaco Star* with pictures I took in Asia. That trip seems a lifetime ago.

Now that I'm stronger, I've allowed a few of my other Texaco friends to come. When I told Bob Lehrman, a writer, that I don't read newspapers or magazines because my bookstand can't hold them, he's appalled. A week later he shows up with a notebook that does fit into my bookstand. He has filled with articles.

He now has the Texaco editorial staff clipping newspaper and magazine pieces for me. Tim Lanigan, the office conservative, even slips in long articles from the *National Review*. I look forward to those notebooks more than they'll ever know.

Clare Ann has come up with a new activity to add to my miseries. She has talked Dr. Schick into recommending that I sit up on the side of the bed with my feet dangling. It's supposed to help my respiration, circulation and sense of balance. If it is so therapeutic, why didn't the marvelous Dr. Schick think of it herself?

What is it with Clare Ann? She gives me as little support as she can, after she sits me up. She knows it terrifies me. I feel I'm going to slip off the mattress and crash to the floor. Laura is afraid of sitting me up, but Clare Ann has bullied her into it. When she does it, she always sits next to me with her arm around my shoulders. She wants to be certain I'm secure.

I asked her tonight to put me in the wheelchair and take me to the window near the elevator. It looks out over the George Washington Bridge. I've had glimpses of the bridge from here with Clare Ann while we're waiting for an elevator, but she's too impatient to wait for me to really look.

Now, I stare at the bridge through the open window. It's as beautiful as ever. Its thick cables swoop down to meet the graceful arc of the roadway. I crossed that bridge twice a day for years. Now I wonder if I'll ever cross it again, ever get to go home.

"What's wrong? Why are you crying?" Laura asks.

I'm thinking of my father, I lie. She won't understand

my being homesick. But mouthing the word father reminds me of that loss and makes me cry more intensely.

I have wept over him at least once every day since his death. Usually I save my tears for Rikki, who is patient and understanding, but sometimes I cry when I'm alone. Dr. Ramsbotham says that it is perfectly normal for a person with a neurological disorder to cry, but I don't think my tears have much to do with my illness.

I'm still biting the air. I wonder if it is connected with Guillain-Barré. It sure is driving Clare Ann nuts. She's always yelling at me to stop and she's even punched me in the arm a few times to let me know that I'm doing it again. I do it unconsciously and I haven't a clue as to why I find it so strangely satisfying.

"Good afternoon sir. How are you today?" Dr. Ramsbotham asks. Okay, I mouth, but he's not even looking for an answer. "I've brought my colleague, Dr. Steinberg, to meet you," he says, introducing, a short, stocky, bearded man. "I've asked him to try to clear up the mystery of why you've developed this habit of biting the air." I didn't know that Clare Ann had told him. I'm embarrassed that he knows about it. It's just a nervous mannerism.

"I've thoroughly reviewed your chart," Dr. Steinberg is saying, "and there's really no mystery. Your biting the air is an after affect of the tranquilizer you had."

Tranquilizer? I've never had a tranquilizer in my life. What tranquilizer? I ask Clare Ann.

"Oh dear, what's he saying?" asks Dr. Ramsbotham. "I'm not good at reading lips, you know."

"Robert's asking what tranquilizer?" Clare Ann tells him.

"The tranquilizer I ordered after you had the sad news about your father. Clare Ann thought you needed something to take your mind off your troubles."

You never told me!

"Robert's saying we never told him," Clare Ann reports.

"He'll stop biting the air on his own." Dr. Steinberg says, ignoring the discussion. "It's just a matter of time."

"That's good news then, isn't it sir?" Dr. Ramsbotham says. "Well, we must go. Good afternoon sir."

Why didn't you say anything about a tranquilizer? I ask Clare Ann angrily. I wouldn't have taken it; I wouldn't have chosen numbness.

"You were very upset then," she says, refusing to discuss it more. I'm outraged that she drugged me without telling me. I'm also infuriated that for weeks she's been hounding me about biting the air and she was the cause.

"You gave it to Bob without telling him?" Rikki asks later.

"Yes," Clare Ann admits.

"How could you have done that?" she demands. "It should have been his decision!"

"I know what's good for him. He needed something."

"I'll discuss this with Dr. Ramsbotham," Rikki says, exasperated.

Dr. Ramsbotham doesn't really understand why Rikki is upset. "Quite right," he says, trying to placate her. "We should have had Mr. Samuels's permission before we proceeded. We'll be sure to ask about medication in the future, won't we?" he asks Clare Ann. She nods in agreement, but I know nothing will change.

Although Clare Ann thinks she's very sensitive, she is often oblivious to how I feel. Every time we go to the therapy floor, she must bring my thick hospital chart with us. She puts it on my lapboard and uses my hands as a paperweight. I hate that. I hate having a part of my body treated like an inanimate object. When I object she doesn't understand.

Seeing the other rehab patients no longer upsets me and their stories fascinate me. There's Enrico, a wealthy, middle-aged businessman from Argentina. In a bizarre accident, the propeller of his own plane hit him in the back. It paralyzed him from the waist down. Enrico is determined to walk again. The therapists have him standing between parallel bars. He wears heavy metal leg braces. Clare Ann admires his grit.

In sharp contrast, there's Joe from the Bronx, supposedly a minor mafioso. He's young, maybe in his late twenties. He has the sensual good looks of a youthful Marlon Brando. A bullet severed Joe's spinal cord. They say he won't tell the cops who shot him.

Like Enrico, he's paralyzed from the waist down, but he isn't sitting much less standing. Because he has bedsores on his butt, he spends his time lying on his stomach on a stretcher. It has wheelchair-type wheels in the front so he can push himself around.

Clare Ann says Joe doesn't try. "It's all attitude, Robert." She's implying, in her usual blunt way, that if my attitude were more like Enrico's and less like Joe's, I'd be standing too. That is totally ridiculous. Joe doesn't have a private duty nurse, but if he did I wish it were Clare Ann. He'd have her rubbed out.

Enrico's wife is throwing a birthday party for him. She's invited all the rehab patients including me. I can't take the invitation seriously. How can I go to a party? I couldn't eat, drink, or talk with anyone. I'd be dying to get back to bed the whole time.

The party is late this afternoon, Clare Ann reminds me after Rikki leaves. I don't want to go, I tell her. We're going, she says. No! The party will be good for me, she argues. Everyone will be disappointed if I don't show up. There's no stopping her.

They've decorated the big therapy room with flowers and crepe paper. Enrico is delighted to see me. He wheels over and introduces his attractive young wife and two young children. "My wife will bring you a plate of food," he says, pointing toward a table covered with cold cuts and salads. I shake my head no. I'm surprised he doesn't realize that I can't really eat.

"Robert already ate," Clare Ann explains, accepting their invitation to get herself some food.

"Would you care for a drink, Robert?" Enrico asks. No, I nod but he misunderstands and has his wife bring me a Scotch on the rocks. I can't lift my arm much less a glass. "I'm going to leave the drink on your lapboard," Clare Ann says when they excuse themselves. "It makes you look more natural." Bourbon would make me look natural. I hate Scotch.

"How, ya doing?" Joe asks, rolling toward me on his stretcher. I nod yes. "I'm glad to see you got a drink." I nod yes again. "How about a cigarette?" he offers, holding out a pack. No, I nod. "Don't smoke, huh?" That's right. Just breathing is enough right now, thank you.

"Mary," he calls, to a pretty, but plump young woman in a low-cut party dress. "This here is Mary, my girlfriend." She reaches out to shake, but both my hands stay firmly on the lapboard, exactly where Clare Ann placed them a half-hour ago. "Mary's a singer," Joe explains, not noticing her embarrassment. I nod. I'm not much of a conversationalist.

Arthur, another patient I've come to recognize, smiles and waves to me. He's a handsome black man in his late sixties or early seventies. They amputated his left leg just below the knee, a complication of diabetes. He's going to be fitted with an artificial leg, but while he's waiting, he's helping the occupational therapists. They're using his skills as a professional carpenter by having him make new equipment. Arthur seems glad to have something useful to do.

There is a real need here for new equipment. I'm always teasing Rhoda, my occupational therapist, about how old the stuff is. We were both shocked when a group of visiting therapists from Harlem Hospital, a city-owned facility, were envious of what we have. I can't imagine what they have.

A friend of Arthur's is softly playing a set of drums in the corner. Arthur's joining him now with a silver trumpet. He's good. They're both good. "Arthur played professionally before he became a carpenter," Clare Ann tells me. I'll bet the drummer did too.

Now Mary, Joe's girl friend, gets up. She's huskily singing "Some of These Days" into a microphone. I can see by the way she's staring at Joe that she loves him, mafia or not, paralyzed or not. There is something enormously moving about this group. They break into "Give My Regards to Broadway," a favorite of my father's, and I struggle to hold back my tears. I want to go back to my bed.

Enrico and his family and the other patients are having a great time. Why shouldn't they? They're all less handicapped than I am. One of the stroke victims is dancing with a nurse. I'm the only one not able to eat and drink.

But my condition is temporary, I remind myself. They're all worse off than I am. The guy with the stroke can't talk. Enrico and Joe will never be normal. I'll make a full recovery. I'm like someone temporarily living in a homeless shelter while waiting for his inheritance to come through.

~

Rhoda Levin, my occupational therapist, knowing I make my living writing, has started me typing. She has my arms hanging from the slings, and a pencil in each of my braces. She puts a portable electric in front of me, and rolls in some paper.

"Niw is the tome..." I type by hitting the keys with the erasers. I think it is remarkably good for the first attempt. I practice some more, delighted with what I can do.

"dear Rlkki," I type. "I love you. you're gnat. love bob xxxxxxxxxxxxxxxxxxxxxxxxxxxxxxxxxxxxxxxxxxxxxxxxx"

I have Clare Ann put the note on my bed so Rikki will see it as soon as she gets here. She's thrilled that I've written something.

I'm at the typewriter again. I want to write to my stepmother. "Dear Louise," I begin. "I am tping this leter muselfy. My arms are up in slings. I feel lik a puppet."

Sudden tears block my vision. The letter makes me sound so pitiful. I want to ask about my father. I want to know exactly what happened to him.

Rikki has only seen me in therapy a couple of times because Clare Ann doesn't want her there. She got Rosemary Schneider, my therapist, to say that she prefers not to have groups of family members in the room when she's working. Rikki isn't a group, but Clare Ann has twisted the message to make it sound as though Rosemary would rather Rikki not visit too often. I don't know how to fight this. It isn't important enough to me to start another battle with Clare Ann. I don't have the energy.

Big news! I hit 940 cc's on my last vital capacity test. Dr. Schick thinks it's close enough to 1,000 cc's to start weaning me from the respirator. They'll have me on the machine less and less each day until I only use it when I sleep. I'll need it then, Dr. Schick says, because my diaphragm still isn't working. Unless she thinks it is, she'll keep me on the machine forever.

I'm spending most of every day off the respirator and I'm finding it difficult. I've become addicted to it just as I was to cigarettes. I even miss its sound when they turn it off.

"Robert, do you know what day July Fourth is?" Clare Ann asks. Does she think I'm simple?

Independence Day, I tell her.

"That's right," she says, "and that's the day we're going to declare your independence from the respirator."

Today's the fourth and I'm off the machine. The room is so quiet without it. Shaun comes by on his afternoon service call but there's no need for him to change the hoses this time. "Soon you won't need me or Nurse Ratched at all," he says.

Laura knew I'd make it. To celebrate, she's brought in a small American flag and tied it to the respirator. When she hooks me up for the night, it's like finally having a cigarette after going all day without one. I welcome the sound of the machine. It's my lullaby. I sleep as if I've been working all day digging ditches.

"I think you're strong enough to try talking," Clare Ann says one morning. She blocks the air escaping from the hole in my trach tube with a white plastic plug. I'm speechless at first because it's all so unexpected.

"Try talking, Robert," she urges impatiently. "Testing, testing, testing," I reply in a very weak voice. I'm half-surprised that I remember how to form words. "That's fantastic!" she says. She summons several floor nurses. "Show them what you can do, Robert."

"Hello, hello," I say faintly.

I'm waiting for Rikki. I have to stay up because if I lie down with the plug in I can't breathe. My ass is killing me. I'm angry with everyone. "What took you so long?" I want to ask when she arrives but instead I manage, "Hello, beautiful."

She hears the words but it is so surprising that at first she doesn't grasp they're from me. "Did you say that?" she asks, confused. She hasn't heard my voice in months.

"You were expecting Pavarotti?" I whisper.

"I wasn't expecting anyone," she smiles, hugging me.

"Mrs. Samuels, please leave the room. I want to put your husband to bed," Clare Ann says. She's late for her lunch because she's been keeping me up so I could talk to Rikki.

"Over and out," are my final words.

Because it's so much harder to breathe without the plug, I save my talking periods to surprise friends. I can only speak a few sentences at a time. I can amaze them by just saying hello. My voice, which is muffled and difficult to understand, doesn't sound like me. Clare Ann says it will return to normal when they remove the trach tube. I hope she's right. Mostly, I still mouth words silently, or spell them out for Rikki and others who don't lip-read.

In all these months I haven't had a bath or a shower, just bed baths. Clare Ann says she is trying to find a mesh-covered stretcher that's used for showers. I'm looking forward to it.

The stretcher is missing. No one knows what happened to it, but Clare Ann has something else we can use. "It's a shower chair," she explains, showing it to me. It looks like a small wheelchair with a toilet seat for a seat. Before I know it, she's jacking me up with the Hoyer lift and, with the help of another nurse, lowering me into it. I'm uncomfortable sitting on pillows in my regular wheelchair. This is agonizing.

"How do you like it?" she asks. I shrug, pretending indifference. She'll be angry if I tell her the truth. She's angry anyway. "You never appreciate anything I do for you! You're never grateful!" She's pushing me down the hall as fast as she can. When we reach the shower room we have to wait. Someone's in it.

Clare Ann is sitting on a bench and I'm on my toilet seat, covered with a sheet. The pain is horrible. If she handed me a gun, and I was strong enough to use it, I'd happily splatter my brains over the ceiling. She's telling me again that I'm the worst patient she's ever had. "You'll never get better because you don't try." Oh God, get this over. The person in the shower is taking all day. Is he singing an entire opera in there? My tailbone feels as if it is being rubbed raw. "You only care about yourself!"

Finally, a little old lady in a robe and clutching a walker comes slowly out. One of the floor nurses is with her. Move it! I silently shout. When she passes, Clare Ann pushes me quickly past her, through the door, smashing my bare foot into a tile wall. The pain actually takes my breath away. I'm crying. "What's wrong now!" she yells at me, her voice echoing off the walls of the small, steamy room.

Foot, I mouth, pain! Oh, Jesus. "Just swallow the pain, Robert! You have to swallow the pain. I got a corn that hurts all the time. I never tell you about that!"

She's spraying me with a hand-held nozzle, being careful not to get water in my open trach. No shower ever felt more wonderful, but it isn't worth the pain. "You want another shower tomorrow?" she asks when I'm settled back in bed. No thanks, I mouth. She's in a rage again. "Whether you want it or not, you're going to have one tomorrow and every day from now on!"

My tailbone burns and my foot still hurts. Can you try again to find the stretcher? I ask. "The stretcher has disappeared," she replies, emphasizing each word, as if I'm simple. "I'm not wasting any more of my time looking for it." She's so stubborn and perverse that I think if she stumbled over it in the hall she'd pretend not to see it.

Because I've lost the natural padding of flesh and fat that once covered my tailbone, every time Rosemary, my physical therapist, puts me on the hard exercise mat, she protects my rear end with a pillow. It isn't helping today. Rosemary rolls me on my side and peeks down the back of my pajama to see why I'm complaining. She finds a raw spot on my coccyx and shows it to Clare Ann. "It's the start of a bed sore," Clare Ann says with alarm.

It didn't happen in bed, I tell her. The shower chair caused it. "That isn't true," she says. "You caused the red spot," she insists. "Every time we position you on your side you complain about your legs being too bent. We've been letting you lie partially on your back and that's what's made this happen! Well, no more. From now on you're staying off your back."

Several days have gone by and Clare Ann can't understand why the sore hasn't healed. She's been putting a salve on it and keeping me on my side. She suspects Laura is letting me lie on my back at night. It's the shower chair, I tell her. It rubs me raw every morning. She refuses to believe me.

Great news! Because Laura happened to mention that Clare Ann plans to take off for a three-day weekend, Rikki's had time to line up my favorite replacement, Kathleen Cunningham, the Irish nurse. As soon as Kathleen starts, I let her know about the shower chair problem. "We'll skip showers this weekend," she says sensibly.

The first thing Clare Ann does when she returns is check the sore. "The new salve worked. It's healed," she says, delighted. That's not why it's better, I tell her. It's because I didn't have any showers while you were away. She tells me I'm wrong. I have no medical training. It's back to the shower chair.

My coccyx again is constantly raw. Some days it is better than others and that makes Clare Ann believe she has solved the problem. Other days it's worse and she blames me. The pain is horrible when I'm in that chair. I complain as much as I dare. It does no good.

More progress. They are planning to remove my stomach tube. They haven't used it for the past couple of weeks, but they wanted to make sure that I could maintain my weight without it. It has held steady at 145. I've not weighed that little since high school.

Taking the tube out doesn't sound difficult. Ever since I've had it, Clare Ann has been scaring me by warning it could accidentally fall out. All that holds it in, she's explained, is its mushroom-shaped end.

Well, I guess she was wrong about it coming out on its own. Three different residents have tried to pull it out but they get scared and back off when they see they're hurting me. "Maybe they'll have to cut it out," Clare Ann says. She's kidding, I hope.

I'm alone watching the news at noon when Dr. Clark, the surgeon, startles me by wandering in unexpectedly "I heard you want the tube out," he says. Yes, I nod, not certain now if I really do. I sure don't want him cutting it out. He draws back the sheet and looks under my hospital gown. I don't see a scalpel in his hands. "All right," he says, grabbing my tube and giving it a big yank. I feel a quick, sharp pain and out it pops.

"That's it," he tells me. "The hole might leak a little at first but it should heal very nicely."

Now I wish I still had the tube. Every meal is unpleasant. Clare Ann is impatient and makes me eat too fast. When food is stuck in my cheeks, my tongue is too weak to remove it. Yesterday, some pieces of overdone hamburger got caught in the back of my throat. When I told Clare Ann, she said it was my imagination.

These days when Burger King asks, "Aren't you hungry?" I want to shout, "Not anymore!"

Clare Ann found a wishbone in my roast chicken dinner (one of the hospital's better dishes). She's taped it over my bed for good luck. She proudly points it out to all my visitors. It's the happiest I've seen her since the day she had my palm read. What next, a voodoo doctor?

Laura is here early. "Robert, I have a surprise for you," she says, her voice filled with anticipation. She's cranking up my bed. I still hate sitting this way. What are you doing? I ask indignantly.

"Just wait," she tells me. She's covering my tray table with a linen napkin. "Remember when I promised you this?" she asks. With a flourish, she presents a still-warm lobster on a fine china plate. She also has a small bottle of chilled white wine and a crystal wine glass. She's even managed a cup of melted butter and a nutcracker. It's what a hospital might serve a movie star in for a facelift.

Where did you get all this, I ask, overwhelmed. She brought it from home, she tells me. She packed everything in a picnic basket and took a taxi to the hospital. What makes it especially touching is that Laura knows nothing about lobsters. She's never eaten or cooked one. The fish market man told her how long to boil it. I have to mouth instructions on how to crack the shell.

"Is it good?" she asks anxiously, after feeding me the first forkful. It's delicious, the best lobster I ever had, I tell her, but in truth it seems rubbery and hard to chew. But I know there's nothing wrong with the lobster. The trouble is my weak mouth and jaw.

She's even remembered to bring a corkscrew. She holds the glass so I can sip the wine. It tastes awful, more like raw alcohol than wine. "Is it okay?" she asks. You try it, I tell her. She doesn't want to; she's on duty. She's such a square! Just a taste, I urge. Finally, she does. Her expression tells me that there's nothing wrong with the wine. It's me, my taste buds. I can't eat or drink most of what she brought but I'm overwhelmed by what she's done.

"Wasn't it nice of Laura to bring you the lobster dinner?" Clare Ann asks in the morning. It certainly was, I reply. I expect her to make fun of Laura, start calling her the lobster nurse or something like that. Instead, she turns on me. "You don't appreciate all we do for you," she yells.

Yes, I do, I reply. Laura is wonderful, I add.

"Remember, you fired her," she reminds me. I'd almost forgotten. "You broke her heart."

She's forgiven me, I answer.

Clare Ann says she and Laura should resign when I'm completely free of the respirator. I should start getting used to living without private duty nurses. I won't have any at the rehab hospital, she points out. The idea of their quitting terrifies me. Except for clicking my tongue, there will be no way for me to call anyone if I need help.

I'll have to do a lot of adjusting for the rehab hospital, Clare Ann continually reminds me. They'll force me to spend all day in my wheelchair. I can't imagine that. I couldn't survive even a whole morning out of bed.

Rehabilitation hospitals teach self-reliance, she adds. If, for example, I fall out of my wheelchair, I'll have to get back by myself, even if it takes hours. "What will you do then?" she asks. I say nothing. I can't crawl an inch much less climb back into a chair. I doubt her, but I'm frightened.

Clare Ann loves celebrities. She remembers every one she's ever seen or met. She never tires of telling me about her conversations with Frank Sinatra when he would call to ask about a famous songwriter she was nursing. Ever since she read that Joseph Heller, the novelist, has Guillain-Barré, she's been comparing us. "I'll bet Heller doesn't ask to go back to bed all the time," she'll say. How does she know? Maybe Heller never gets out of bed.

We don't have to wonder about Heller any longer. *People* magazine has a major story about him. It calls Guillain-Barré a very serious illness. I'm surprised to read that because Clare Ann always acts as if it is not much worse than a cold.

Although Heller and I got sick at about the same time, he's already completed rehab and is home in East Hampton on Long Island, working on his next book. He's still very weak and spends much of his time in a wheelchair, but he's walking!

"He must be a marvelous patient," Clare Ann tells me pointedly, as if that had anything to do with his recovery. He had a less severe case than mine, I reply.

"Why do you say that?"

He never even needed a respirator, I point out.

"You think a respirator is so terrible?" she asks.

The magazine reports that Heller and I have had some of the same experiences. He also wasn't able to sleep in the beginning. A psychiatrist told him that it was fear that kept him awake. I wonder if that's why I couldn't sleep.

He too had private duty nurses, but his experience with his main one was not like mine. She's his girlfriend now and she's living with him. This draws no comment from Clare Ann, but it shocks the prudish Laura. It was very unprofessional of Heller's nurse to become romantically involved, she says. He was divorcing his wife when he got sick, I point out. It doesn't matter to her. I wonder what I would have done if I had been living alone when this happened. I couldn't have gotten through this without Rikki.

Heller had only one EMG test. I can't remember how many I've had. He told *People* how horribly painful it was. When a doctor wanted to test him a second time, Heller's best friend asked who would benefit from it. The doctor admitted the test wouldn't help Heller. His friend told the doctor to forget it.

I have to get completely off the respirator soon, Clare Ann says. The summer is slipping by and I should have been in a rehabilitation hospital by now.

Laura is holding me up, Clara Ann says, because she's afraid to have me sleep without the respirator. Laura is afraid of Clare Ann but she's even more afraid of something bad happening to me. "He's been sleeping off the respirator when I'm at lunch and he ain't dead yet," Clare Ann tells her. "Look, if you're scared, just sit in here all night and watch him sleep."

Laura tries, but she's so nervous she's continually shining a flashlight in my face to check my breathing. I can't sleep through that.

If I really wanted to go to a rehab hospital and recover, I'd pretend to sleep through the flashlight, Clare Ann tells me. "You have to convince Laura that you don't need the machine." But I don't know if that's true. Dr. Schick still says my diaphragm isn't working, I remind her.

"Jesus H. Christ! You want to stay here the rest of your life?" I don't answer but I think bad as it is, it's still better than lying like a beached jellyfish on the floor of a rehabilitation hospital if I fall out of my wheelchair.

Dr. Schick has come up with still another gadget. It's a sensor that will sound an alarm if I stop breathing. That should allow me to sleep without worry, she says.

Laura's very mechanical, good with devices like this, so it might work. She positions the sensor on my neck, near my trach opening. "Try holding your breath," she says. As soon as I do, the sensor, which they developed to guard against sudden infant crib death, buzzes like a cheap electric alarm clock.

It's been two nights now and the sensor hasn't let me have much rest. The trouble is that I breathe irregularly when I sleep, causing the alarm to sound. Clare Ann is exasperated. She thinks we should forget the sensor. "Everyone misses an occasional breath when they're asleep. Haven't you ever slept with anyone?" she asks, mortifying Laura with the question.

I've decided, when the time comes, I'll go to the Helen Hayes Rehabilitation Hospital. It's in the suburbs, nearer our house than any of the others. Although the state runs it, everyone here says its first rate. A doctor from Helen Hayes has examined me. They'll be happy to admit me, he said, once I'm off the respirator.

Rikki would rather have me at the Rusk Institute. She argues it's the best in the world, but I have my doubts. I've overheard nurses here say the atmosphere at Rusk is so loose that the employees openly smoke marijuana. That's all I need. I also remember Candy, one of my first nurses, talking about her patient who had gotten bedsores in a "world famous rehabilitation hospital." I'm sure it was Rusk.

Heller had nothing but praise for Rusk in the *People* article, but I don't trust what he says. He's famous and famous people are treated differently everywhere they go.

"You know when people leave they usually give their nurse a gift," Clare Ann tells me.

Yes, I reply. She doesn't have to remind me. Rikki gave both her and Laura nice presents at Christmas. I'm sure she wouldn't have forgotten. "I don't want something just for myself. What would be nice would be for Mrs. Samuels to bring in cold cuts and salads, and the floor nurses could have a party."

That's a good idea, I tell her. She's constantly asking the floor nurses to help her with the Hoyer lift. Generally,

they're a good crew and I like them. The cold cuts will allow
her to play Lady Bountiful, the Big Shot, but what do I care.

Rikki cares. "I have never been so manipulated by
anyone in my life," she says when I tell her. "We should give
her nothing."

"She's terrible but she's done a lot for me," I say in my
weak little voice. We're in the solarium and I have the plug in.

"She's making $150 a day. If she wants to throw a
party, she can buy her own cold cuts. I don't want to get her
anything."

"Look, I don't want any more trouble with her. The
cold cuts can also be our way of thanking the floor nurses. I
want you to do this for me."

"I'll do it only if you insist."

"I insist," I tell her.

~

Miss Rosenberg, my hospital social worker, has been
checking into my transfer to a rehabilitation hospital and
has made a terrible discovery— my insurance will cover only
four weeks of my stay there. The rest, $200 a day at Helen
Hayes (least expensive of all the rehab hospitals), we'll be
expected to pay for ourselves.

I'm stunned. We haven't had to pay any medical bills
since I first arrived. Rikki had to come up with $300 a day for
the nurses in the beginning but they've reimbursed us that.
Until now, my Texaco insurance has taken care of everything
else. Miss Rosenberg, a sad-eyed young woman, is very
sympathetic but she tells us that she can't do more for us.

My stay at the rehab hospital could take many weeks,
even several months. We have some savings and we'll be able

to cover it for a while but eventually it will wipe us out. The house and everything else we own will go.

"The important thing is that you make a complete recovery, not the house," Rikki says, trying to make me feel better, but I can see she's upset too. I know I'll recover, but I don't want us to be impoverished for the rest of our lives. We are both having trouble sleeping because of this.

Dr. Ramsbotham is trying to help us. He's looking into the possibility of my remaining here on the rehab floor instead of moving to a rehab hospital. That way the insurance company would continue to pick up the tab. I hope we can do it.

It won't work. No matter what I do, whether I stay here or not, after four weeks as a rehab patient I'll lose my insurance coverage. Dr. Ramsbotham couldn't be more sympathetic. I think the $200 a day we'll have to pay bothers him particularly because he's English and in England all this would be free.

"Finances should be the last thing on your mind," says Laura, the Republican, when I tell her why I can't sleep. "You can worry about money when you're up walking around," she continues. "Right now just concentrate on getting well."

Why should anyone in a rich country like this have to agonize over medical bills? I ask angrily.

"Are you for socialized medicine?" she asks, shocked. Sometimes I wonder if she lives in a cave.

Yes, I tell her. I'm also for free college educations and decent social security retirement incomes. I even think government should do more to help the poor. Does that make me a Communist?

Clare Ann, who is a liberal Democrat, can't understand why I'm worried about money. She never is. She owns almost nothing, has no savings and borrows for every unexpected expense. She once had to borrow several thousand dollars from a bank to pay off a pile of parking tickets she had ignored. She found that so many people owe large sums for old tickets in New York City that the loan officer didn't blink. To her, this was hilarious.

Laura is taking a week's vacation. Where are you going? I ask. Cape Cod? The Jersey shore? No place. She'll rest at her apartment. That's so Laura.

How can you leave me when you're in the middle of weaning me from the respirator? I ask.

"I have to get away," she says tensely. She's lined up Wilma Cross to take her place. I haven't had Wilma as a nurse, but I know who she is. She seems fine, but I fear all new nurses.

I thought Clare Ann would be furious with Laura for taking off, but instead she's delighted. "Wilma has weaned a lot of people off respirators. She'll have you sleeping without it before the week is out," she predicts. I don't believe it.

This is Wilma's first night. "How you doing?" she asks coming in the door. She's a big, buxom, motherly type. Like Pearl, the nurse who almost killed me, her race is difficult to pinpoint, but unlike Pearl, she inspires confidence.

"Clare Ann wants me to sit you up and let your legs dangle," she says. Jesus, I hate that. Oh, oh, she's pulling back the covers. I thought she was talking about doing it later. I'm scared shitless. I don't know this lady.

I'm sitting on the side and she's next to me with one big brown arm around my shoulders. I'm leaning against her, in the deep valley her weight has pushed in the mattress. I couldn't slip away from her if I tried. "Clare Ann told me it scares you to sit like this," she says with a trace of the Caribbean in her voice. "I hope you're not scared now. I won't let you go," she adds unnecessarily, giving me a big squeeze and a big laugh.

"Clare Ann wants me to try to get you off the respirator," Wilma continues, still holding me tightly. "She told me Laura hasn't been able to do it. I can understand that. I've had that trouble too. You get too sensitive when you've been taking care of one patient for a long time. Some things are easier for strangers to do. Will you let me try?" Yes, I nod.

She's changed my gown, washed and suctioned me. I'm ready for sleep. "I'll be sitting right here," Wilma promises. "If you stop breathing I'll wake you right away and get you back on the respirator. Just relax and don't worry. I know you can do it."

She's left the light on in the bathroom and the door is slightly ajar. In the dim light, I see her sitting in the room's one comfortable chair. I know if I need her she'll be there.

I sleep, and then wake, my left side aching as usual. She's up at my first click. "Want to be turned?" she asks. Yes, I nod, and she turns me. "You're doing real well, honey." I don't worry; I have no fear. The night stretches on and I force myself not to think of what's happening or I'll be too excited to sleep.

It's morning. I've spent my first night without a respirator in almost nine months. "You did great," Wilma tells me as she gets ready to leave. "I don't know another patient who ever done so good."

I'm anxious to see Clare Ann. Despite myself, I want to please her. "I'll talk to you in the nurses' lounge," I hear her tell Wilma.

The wait for Clare Ann seems endless. Too bad I couldn't have kicked the respirator sooner. It seems so easy now. Clare Ann should be overjoyed. We shouldn't have any conflicts today. Here she comes. Christ, why is she scowling?

"You're pretty damned pleased with yourself, ain't you?" she asks. Yes, I nod. "Well, you shouldn't be. If it wasn't for

Wilma, you'd never be off the machine."

Don't I get any credit, I ask.

"No, you don't get any credit," she says nastily. "You should have done this weeks ago. You could be in a rehab program now."

She won't praise me, but she's bragging about me to everyone. Does she think that if she's nice to me it will spoil me and I'll give up? "Robert's been without the machine for more than almost thirty-six hours," she tells Dr. Ramsbotham when he makes his afternoon visit.

"That's remarkable," he says, genuinely astonished. "Dr. Schick will be surprised. She didn't expect that so soon." She didn't expect it at all I want to say. When will I start rehab? I ask.

"We'll have to observe you several weeks before you go anywhere," he answers.

I've been without the respirator for three days. Dr. Schick has finally come to see me. Did she stay away because she's embarrassed? She's listening to my chest with her double-headed stethoscope. "I'm glad you're off the machine," she says. I'm too polite to ask her how I'm able to breathe at night without a functioning diaphragm. She offers no explanation. Clare Ann says nothing.

"How tall are you?" Dr. Schick asks.

Six feet, I tell her. She looks at me strangely.

"You may have shrunk," she says.

I'm in a wheelchair. How can you tell?

"People can lose as much as two inches when they're in bed for months," she explains. My height was about the only thing I liked about my looks. Now she tells me I might be shorter! Jesus, I don't want to think about that.

Clare Ann and Laura will continue caring for me until I go to Helen Hayes. Clare Ann has finally realized it would be dangerous to leave me dependent on floor nurses. I still need frequent suctioning and I'm still not able to press the call button for help.

Both my nurses are planning long vacations after I leave. With their twelve-hour shifts, they've earned enough money not to have to work for months. My illness hasn't been bad for everyone. It's made some people rich. I don't resent it, but I'm thinking that if everyone stayed well until they died, millions would be unemployed. But I'm sure medical professionals don't want people to be sick. When I was a police reporter, I didn't sit around hoping for a juicy murder, but I didn't mind at all if there was one on my watch.

You develop a professional detachment when dealing with tragedy. It's the mind's natural defense. I can remember pretending to be sympathetic when interviewing people who had just learned a loved one had been murdered or killed in a plane crash. I felt as if I were watching a movie.

Occasionally, reality would break through. Early one beautiful spring day, a dog walker discovered a young woman's body in a partially opened car trunk on Riverside Drive. By the time I arrived, the cops knew she was a victim of a drug overdose, something so common it didn't even rate a paragraph in the paper. The detectives were standing around in the cool morning sunlight chatting with a few reporters, guessing that someone who had been with her had probably panicked and dumped the body there.

Through the open trunk, I could see the back of the dead girl. Her sweater had ridden up, exposing about six inches of bare back. There was something about it, maybe the shape of the muscles around her spine that reminded me of Rikki. I had to keep myself from running over and trying to see her face. I was filled with dread, but it couldn't be Rikki. She was home taking care of Charlie. Even later, after I had talked with her on the phone, I had the feeling that something awful had happened. Of course, something awful had happened. It just hadn't happened to someone I loved.

For a while, I understood that the stories I was covering were about real people, but that feeling wore off. The people in my stories had to live forever with their tragedy, while I went home at the end of my shift.

Well, now it's my turn. I'm the one who stays. Even Rikki goes home. I never get a break. I'm not complaining about Rikki. She does everything anyone could do for me. She's the only one who sees my darker side. To everyone else, I'm amazingly happy. I'm even mostly cheerful when I'm alone, but when Rikki and I are by ourselves in the solarium, I often break down. I can't spend the rest of my life like this, I sob. "Things are getting better," she reminds me. "You're going to make a full recovery."

The solarium is my place to cry, my little turret of tears. Everything makes me weep. I'll see a cabin cruiser going up the Hudson on a sparkling Saturday morning and I'll burst into tears, remembering the small boat we once had. Any thought of my father devastates me.

If someone else visits the solarium, Rikki quickly dries my tears so they won't see. We've become friendly with a family from Beirut. Doctors are operating on a relative of theirs who has a brain tumor. These people are Muslims but very modern, urbane, and charming. I'd love to have met them in Beirut before that city went insane. There are wonderful people everywhere. I still have a whole life to live.

~

It is the repeat of a nightmare—the doctor with the Van Dyke is pushing needles into me for my final EMG test. Dr. Ramsbotham says the results will give him a baseline to use when I come back. He expects me to return voluntarily for years so he can periodically test me. I'll be cooperative this one last time, but he's out of his goddamn mind if he thinks I'll ever be back.

The zaps start and so do my tears. I don't have to take this! It has nothing to do with getting better. Heller only went through it once and he's already walking around, going to parties in the Hamptons and working on a book. Stop! Stop! I mouthed, shaking my body as violently as I can.

"You want me to quit?" the Van Dyke asks. Yes, yes, I nod. "Let me get Dr. Ramsbotham. This test is for him."

Dr. Ramsbotham is unavailable. He's gone somewhere for a meeting. The Van Dyke is disconnecting me. He doesn't care if I take the test or not. I'm back on the stretcher, on the elevator. I can't stop the tears. I wanted to do everything they asked, anything that might get me better sooner, but this was too much. It won't make me better.

"What are you crying about? It's all over," Clare Ann asks disgustedly, but I sob until I'm safely back in the room.

Are you pleased I stopped the test? I ask her. She obviously is but she won't admit it. "I told you before that you could refuse," is all she'll say. Why do I care about her opinion? The hell with what she thinks. I'm very relieved and pleased with myself now.

"I wish you would reconsider," Dr. Ramsbotham is saying. He has spilled something on his clownish, purple tie. As he speaks, I notice the curly grey hair coming out of his nose and ears. He should braid them together. How can I listen to such a ridiculous-looking person? "I can reschedule it for tomorrow." No, never! "Oh, dear, what's he saying?" he asks Rikki.

"He's telling you that he doesn't want any more EMG tests," she says sharply.

"Oh, dear! Perhaps, sir, you'll feel differently tomorrow.

I'll ask again." Go ahead and ask, I think, but I'll never change my mind. Never!

As I work on the mat with Rosemary Schneider the next day, Dr. Schick is watching. Rosemary puts my left leg in a sling that hangs from ceiling hooks. I swing the leg back and forth while she goes off to help another patient.

"I don't blame you for stopping the test," Dr. Schick says, sitting on the edge of my mat and patting my hand. "You were very upset then, but you know you'll have to take it eventually." No, I tell her by shaking my head. Why does she care? She doesn't need the results.

"I've always admired your intelligence, Bob," she purrs seductively. "I'm sure you understand that the information from the EMG is vital." Like what? I ask. "Without the results I can't guarantee you won't have a heart attack. You'll take it again, won't you?" No, I tell her by shaking my head vigorously.

She's furious with me, but she's trying to hide it, struggling to regain her Asian cool. "Won't you at least reconsider?" Yes, I nod, knowing I won't but wanting her to go away and leave me alone. She's a goddamn liar, using fear to try to force me to change my mind. There's nothing wrong with my heart. I must have had fifty EKG's since I first got sick. All the results were normal.

Today we're going outside. I haven't been out all summer, Clare Ann says with surprise. "It's creepy to always want to stay in," she adds. She won't listen to any more excuses. Before I know it, I'm down the elevator, through the front door and onto the steep, perilous sidewalk. One slip by her and I'm over the edge. Rikki, unaware of my terror, is practically skipping with excitement.

It's late afternoon, bathing everything in a magical, golden light. If Rembrandt had painted Washington Heights, it would look like this. I had forgotten that an ordinary street could be so beautiful. Now that we're on the flat sidewalk, I'm no longer frightened. We've reached a grassy, park-like area that runs between two buildings. "You want to stop here?" Clare Ann asks. Sure, this will be fine. She takes the white plastic plug that hangs from my neck like a crucifix and pushes it into my trach.

"Testing, testing," I say, making the same joke I make each time she plugs me in. Clare Ann moves to a bench some distance away and lights a cigarette. Rikki sits at my feet and lights one too.

"If we'd known we'd be here you could have brought Ruffy," I tell her. "He could have run around," I add, my eyes misting over at the thought.

"You forget how old he is. He doesn't run around much anymore. I'll bring him with me when you're at Helen Hayes," she promises. "That's just next week, right after Labor Day," she reminds me.

"We won't be able to afford his Alpo once I'm there," I wisecrack.

~

Everything is ready for my transfer. "Have you ordered the cold cuts for Clare Ann's party?" I ask.

"No and I don't want to."

"What do you mean? I thought we agreed." My voice is little more than a whisper.

"What right does she have to tell us what to get her?" Rikki demands, in a louder voice. I look quickly to see if Clare Ann has heard but she's buried her nose, as usual, in *The New York Times*.

"I just want to leave without having any more trouble

with her." My volume is fading from the effort of talking. Breathing is suddenly difficult.

"Do you need the plug out?" Rikki asks.

"Yes."

We're back in the room. On the way, we ran into a male nurse friend of Clare Ann's. Thank God that he took over and pushed me up the dangerous sidewalk at the entrance.

"Do you really insist that I get the cold cuts for that bitch?" Rikki asks when we're alone. Yes. "Then I will," she says, gathering her things to leave. She's too angry to kiss me goodbye.

Dr. Ramsbotham is making a rare morning visit. He hasn't completely given up on changing my mind about having another EMG. "I would very much like you to come in every six months," he says, and I nod as if I think that's a fantastic idea.

He's looking at me seriously and sympathetically. "On the basis of my EMG studies," he's suddenly saying, "I believe you'll make a substantial recovery. By that I mean you'll regain about eighty-five percent of the strength in your trunk but less in your extremities." He's rattling off more percentages, but I'm having a hard time following him. It's like dreaming about odds on horses that might run next week at a track you're not planning to visit.

"You'll be ambulatory," he continues, "but you'll probably need a cane or crutches. The weakness in your hands will make it difficult for you to, ah, say, hold on while standing in a bus. At some time, sir, you might consider surgery to permanently set your hands and feet in functional positions."

Everyone has talked about a complete recovery, a full recovery. No one has mentioned anything less. Will I walk? I ask, stunned.

"Nurse, I think Mr. Samuels is trying to say something."

"He's asking if he'll walk."

"Yes, I told you you'll be ambulatory. I'm quite certain of that. Do you have any more questions, sir?" I'm shaking my head no. I just want him to leave.

He's gone now and Clare Ann is leaning over the bed, talking to me intently. "He doesn't know anything for sure," she's saying fiercely. "If you work hard in therapy you'll do well. You'll recover. All my Guillain-Barré patients have made full recoveries. Some were worse off than you."

I want to believe her but how can I? She has no scientific basis for anything she says. She believes in palm readers and chicken bones. She has three wishbones over my bed right now. She'd call for a witch doctor if one were available. But damn it, she was right about my being able to breathe off the respirator and the marvelous Dr. Schick was wrong.

My hands will have no strength, I tell her.

"That's not what he said, Robert. He said you would have trouble holding on in a bus. Jesus H. Christ, even I have trouble with that. I have to wrap my arm around the pole. So what if you have do that too. Remember, he doesn't know for sure if that will happen. Work hard in therapy and don't worry about what he said. You'll make a full recovery."

She's right. I know she's right. What was that stuff he was saying about having my hands and feet surgically fixed in position? Do they really do that to people? Christ, it sounds barbaric. I'll never allow that to happen to me. My myelin is re-growing. I'm getting better. Clare Ann is right—I'll make a full recovery.

This is my last full day here. I've said goodbye to my therapists and the other patients on the rehab floor. They're disappointed that I won't be moving in with them. I'm going to Helen Hayes, Clare Ann explained, because it is closer to my home. She can't tell them that the therapy there will be better than they are getting here.

I'm a little less anxious about a rehab hospital than I was. When Clare Ann was away, I asked Rosemary, who once worked in one, about the rules. She said the staff will be sympathetic and I won't have to stay in a wheelchair all day if I'm in pain.

I wonder if Clare Ann made that up as a way of making me sit up longer, or maybe she really thinks they run rehab hospitals like Nazi boot camps. Did she ever visit one? Well, I don't have to think about her much longer. Tomorrow I'll be gone. I just want to leave without any more trouble. I'll die if Rikki doesn't bring the cold cuts. Jesus, just let me out of here.

Rikki is late. She was supposed to bring the food in early. Clare Ann is putting me into bed, getting ready to go to lunch. Is she really going out? Has she forgotten her party?

"I'm here," Rikki calls through the closed door. She must have brought the food.

"This is the last noon time I'll be putting you back to bed," says Clare Ann. She's been making remarks like this all morning, as if today is some great sentimental occasion. "How are you?" she asks Rikki cheerily as she opens the door.

"I'm fine," Rikki replies stiffly, adding, without pause, "The damn cold cuts you wanted are in the nurses' lounge." Oh, Rikki, why did you have to say that?

"Cold cuts? What are you talking about? I didn't ask for any cold cuts," says Clare Ann, her tone rising like a space rocket heading for the moon.

"Sure you did. You asked Bob for them weeks ago. You wanted to have a party for the other nurses."

"I never asked for anything," she says, marching out of the room.

I'm angry, embarrassed, mortified. Couldn't you have simply given her the cold cuts? I ask. We could have pretended it was our idea.

"But it wasn't our idea—it was hers. I couldn't let her get away with manipulating us again. I resent being told to buy a present to show my appreciation, particularly when I'm told exactly what present to buy by the person who is going to receive it. We don't owe her anything. She was paid well for every shift she worked. She wasn't doing us any favors!"

It's late in the afternoon. Clare Ann has closed the door to my room. I'm really in for it. "I didn't ask for cold cuts," she's insisting. I've never seen her so upset. Maybe she lies to herself.

"I don't expect presents from patients." Suddenly I'm infuriated. I'm glad Rikki was so blunt.

"Robert, did I ask for anything?" she asks. Yes, I tell her. You did.

"You know that's not true!" she says with anguish. "I don't care about presents at all. When I get home I'm throwing out what your wife gave me for Christmas!"

It's late. This may be the last time I ever see Clare Ann. She has her reindeer sweater and her belted blue trench coat over her nurse's uniform "Well, good luck, Robert," she tells me woodenly. It's been a tough day for her. Her green eyes are dull and sunken. She looks completely exhausted. "I'm sure you'll make a full recovery. Work hard at Helen Hayes. Too bad our last day couldn't have been more pleasant."

Goodbye, I tell her. Too bad all our days couldn't have been more pleasant.

Laura is feeding me small pieces of rare roast beef, a left over from Clare Ann's party. At least I'm enjoying the food, I joke.

"You may think what happened was funny, but Clare Ann's feelings were really hurt."

Yes, I know.

"She told me she never asked you for the cold cuts."

Well, she did.

"Are you sure?"

Do you think I'd make that up?

"You really don't like her, do you?"

No, I don't.

"You forget all she did for you," she reminds me. "She got you therapy before anyone thought you were ready. She found you a wheelchair and she pushed to have you weaned off the respirator. If it wasn't for her, you still might not have had your first shower."

That's all true, I admit. Few of the nurses I had were as capable as Clare Ann, and none were as driven, but I would have been better off with some others. Kathleen Cunningham, the Irish nurse, for one, is every bit as good as Clare Ann and she wouldn't have made my life such hell. So what if everything happened a couple of weeks later. Getting in a wheelchair sooner hasn't speeded my recovery. Nobody, including Clare Ann, can make myelin grow faster.

"She's not all bad," says Laura, loyal to the end.

I never said she was. She is a good nurse, she's given me faith in my recovery, but she was very hard on me, cruel in fact.

"She really cared for you."

She had funny ways of showing it.

"Robert, someday you'll look back on all this and remember it differently. You'll be grateful to Clare Ann."

No, I won't, but I am grateful to you, and I always will be. You made it possible for me to endure her. If I'd had two Clare Ann's, I would have ended up with a nervous breakdown, I tell her.

"You're exaggerating."

I don't think so.

Laura must get me ready for the ambulance. She's like a young mother anxiously sending her first born off to nursery school. Will the ambulance have a suction machine? How will the attendants get me from my bed to their stretcher?

She doesn't want me to have the plug in when I travel. I want to be able to tell the attendants if I have a problem. I also want them to understand that I'm able to speak, that I'm not in a coma. It would be inviting trouble to have the plug in for such a long time, Laura says. Finally, we compromise. I'll wear it until I'm in the ambulance. That way I'll be able to talk with the attendants before we get going.

They're here, right on time, and Laura is rushing around gathering up things. Unlike her, they're very calm. Yes, they have a suction machine and they both know how to use it. They expertly slide me from the bed to the stretcher. It's so narrow I barely fit. I was only 145 yesterday when they weighed me. That's almost sixty pounds less than when I arrived. How did I fit on the stretcher then?

Goodbye, room. They're rolling me out into the hall; we're passing the nursing station. Some of the floor nurses are kissing me. All of them helped me one time or another.

"Come back and see us when you're well," says Mrs. Roberts, a dignified Jamaican nursing aide who always told me I was her boy friend.

"You'll have the first dance," I promise.

I want to linger but we are already on an elevator. We're going through a back door. The ambulance is a Dodge van. "I thought you'd bring a Cadillac," I tell them. "I'm disappointed."

"They haven't built Cadillac ambulances for a long time," one of the attendants explains, smiling. "It's all vans now. They're roomier and cheaper."

"Cheaper? My insurance is paying you guys a hundred and fifty bucks to drive me the thirty miles to Helen Hayes. We could have hired a limo for a lot less."

"Limos don't have stretchers and suction machines, Robert," says Laura.

"Good point." They're fastening my stretcher to the floor of the van so it won't slide around. Laura's climbed in with us. She pulls my plug. The attendants know that one click of my tongue means yes and two means no. A series of clicks signal that I'm having a problem and need their attention.

"I'll be up to see you after you get settled," says Laura, her eyes shimmering with tears. For a moment, I think she'll kiss me goodbye, but that wouldn't be professional. "Don't fight with the nurses at Helen Hayes," she calls as one of the attendants closes the door.

"You all set, sir?" the driver asks, starting the motor.

Yes, I tell him by clicking my tongue once.

October 2011

I wrote most of this book in the 1980s, when my memories were fresh. That is how I am able to recount my experiences and emotions of more than 30 years ago.

I had put my manuscript aside, but at the urging of my son Charlie and Grace Radin, a friend who had read it years ago, I picked it up again. I was delighted to find the writing still seemed vivid and real.

I don't know if a patient today would have the same experiences that I had at Nyack Hospital and Columbia-Presbyterian Hospital (now New York-Presbyterian Hospital). I hope not. I hope both hospitals have improved.

Like most people, I hadn't realized that U.S. hospital patients are in more peril than motorists on the nation's highways. A landmark 1999 report found that medical mistakes cause as many as 98,000 deaths, and more than one million injuries a year. By contrast, accidents on America's roads that year killed some 41,000 people and injured some 3 million.

I am very lucky to have survived. Some preventable in-hospital medical errors seem easy to correct but aren't for reasons that defy explanation. For example, study after study reports that doctors spread infections by not washing their hands.

Plasmapheresis now is a standard treatment for Guillain-Barré Syndrome. It "lessens the severity of the illness and accelerates the recovery in most patients," reports the National Institute of Neurological Disorders and Stroke. In 1981, when it could have done me some good, plasmapheresis was still "experimental." However, even then my doctors knew they should do it early if it were to work at all. I find it inexcusable that they delayed my treatments until my family insisted they begin.

Nothing Clare Ann told me about rehabilitation hospitals was true. The staff does not make you stay in your wheelchair all day and they would rush to help anyone who fell on the floor. The social worker, who had caused us many sleepless nights, also had been wrong. My insurance had no limit on its coverage for in-hospital rehab treatment.

I found Helen Hayes Hospital to be a very depressing place. It had a large nursing staff but it didn't want to do much. It neglected basic hygiene, bathing patients only once a week. My rehab sessions there were spotty and the food was abominable. I understand that conditions there have improved enormously.

After I was there for just two weeks, my doctor invited me and Rikki to what they said was a routine meeting. At its start, she told us that she planned to discharge me soon because Guillain-Barré patients don't improve after one year. We were stunned. It contradicted everything we had heard and read. Fortunately, I was able to transfer to the Rusk Institution of Rehabilitation Medicine.

Rusk doctors had no timetable for Guillain-Barré. The atmosphere there was upbeat; the staff, filled with wonderful and warm characters. It had, in the words of Kristjan Ragnarsson, one of my doctors, "the spirit of a winning football team." Daily showers in well-padded chairs were part of the routine.

I grew stronger. I began feeding myself and pushing my own wheelchair. I also started moving my hands. My progress so impressed one doctor that without bothering with any respiratory test he pulled out my tracheotomy tube. I was elated, but later that day my physical therapist noticed I was turning blue. Without the tube to help me breathe, I had developed severe pneumonia. It was another life-threatening medical blunder.

The Rusk doctors asked Clement Marks, an internist and respiratory specialist from the New York University Medical Center, which is next door, to take over. In less than a week, the pneumonia was gone. It was several more years before doctors finally removed the trach tube, and another year before they sewed up the hole in my throat.

I had expected to stay at Rusk until I started walking. The occupational therapist the hospital sent to look over our old house reported that it would be nearly impossible to make it wheelchair friendly. They suggested that we add an accessible wing. Knowing it would take forever just to win zoning approval for any construction, I was sure I'd be on my feet before we had permission to break ground.

That was fine with me, but not with Rusk's doctors. They couldn't wait all that time for us to start building. They felt I'd make as much progress at home as I would in the hospital. I could continue my therapy as an outpatient. Others needed my bed more than I did.

We were fearful, angry and resentful. They were forcing us to sell the home we'd loved and lived in for fifteen years. Rikki looked frantically for a place that could accommodate a wheelchair. She seriously considered an old elementary school and a shuttered gas station. Just as it seemed hopeless, we found a nearly completed modern house, only a mile from the old one.

After one look, we agreed to buy it. The architect was someone we had known. He started designing entrance ramps and a modified bathroom for the house. Insurance paid for the changes and promised to cover home nursing care. Rikki phoned Kathleen Cunningham, the nurse we both liked. She lived not far from us and yes, she'd love to become my fulltime home care nurse.

Now we were excited about my coming home and so were our friends. They told Rikki not to hire movers. In a torrential moving day rainstorm, about 50 of them used a rented truck to haul all we owned in to our new house. They worked like Amish farmers at a barn raising.

The next day the sun shone brightly and the same friends were at our new house for a party to welcome me home. It was April 17, 1983, one year, four months and fifteen days after I first became ill. I had survived and I was certain that it was just a matter of time until I made a full recovery.

The realization that it was not to happen came on gradually. I still cannot walk or make full use of my hands.

Rikki and I remained together for another 10 years and then we separated and divorced. I had adjusted very well to my disabilities. I had no choice. It was much harder for her. She had a choice. Both of us found other partners and are happy today. We seldom see each other, but we are friendly when we do. We share a wonderful son, an amazing granddaughter and many memories.

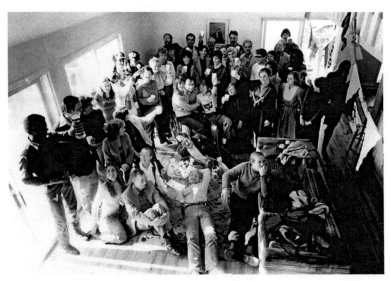

The large group of friends who welcomed me home to our
new house. Sally Savage photo.

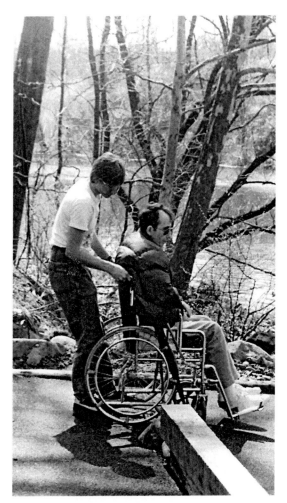

Charlie shows me around the outside of the new house.
Sally Savage photo.

CPSIA information can be obtained at www.ICGtesting.com
Printed in the USA
BVOW021354270312

286189BV00001B/21/P